C.U.R.E.
Cultivating Unlimited
Rejuvenating Energy

The definitive method to reverse the process of disease and regain health, life and vitality

Rosanne Calabrese AP

Table of Contents

"The human body is not only capable, but also innately designed to heal itself. It is us who thwart that process with the habits that we form."

Rosanne Calabrese

Dedication

Any endeavor we undertake is not shouldered alone. Whether it is someone by your side or behind the scenes, there is always a person who has inspired, supported, or challenged you to accomplish great things. In my case, there have been two people in my life that have done this and I can truly say that I would not have walked in this world of healing or written this book if not for them. It is from my heart and with deep gratitude that I dedicate this book to them.

First off, I want to thank my mother Sadie Calabrese. She is no longer with us in the physical form, yet she remains in my heart, my soul, and my thoughts every day of my life. My mother was told that she would die in her twenties (she lived to be 88 years old), that she would never have children (my brother was born just before mom turned 38 and I was born one week after she turned 39), and that she would have heart problems due to the rheumatic fever she battled in her teens (she never took a single prescription drug for her heart and walked a mile just a few months before she passed away). Mom always encouraged me to follow my dreams. She felt that I could do anything. She dreamt of joining the WAC (Woman's Army Corps) during World War II, but the rheumatic fever that she contracted in her early teens stopped her from pursuing that dream. Nevertheless, any time I would come to her with a new career path (fitness instructor, fire fighter, and finally Acupuncture Physician) mom would be so enthusiastic, rooting me on to "go for it!" Mom became vegan at 70, went to the gym four days a week, and could outdo anyone in the kitchen! Her support throughout my life has given me the courage to embrace change and run with it.

Next, I am forever grateful to my husband Anthony Serpico for never, ever, ever losing his faith in me and my ability to heal from Graves' disease. He believes 100% in my ability to help others in their healing journey. Anthony insists on calling me "doctor" (I'm still not sure whether it's a compliment or an insult) and feels that the work that I do is one of the highest levels of healing on our planet. He is the love of my life and my inspiration for all that is fitness, health, and wellbeing. He's also been vegan for 24+ years and flaunts a 54-year-old body that ROCKS even more than a 25 year old's! Anthony is my inspiration for always striving to do better, work harder, and most importantly be happy and take care of myself. He challenged himself during my detoxification process by spending 12 weeks on fruits, vegetables, and herbs alongside me. He kept me on track and true to the process with lots of love. I am truly blessed to have such a wonderful husband and partner in life.

Preface

Who doesn't want to write a book sometime in their life? It was during my high school psychology class that I first discovered I enjoyed writing. My teacher instructed the class to keep a journal that only we would read. We were to jot down all of our happy times, sad times, challenges, and the emotions associated with them. Years later, in my college creative writing class, I was encouraged by my professor to pursue a degree in English. I quickly dismissed her suggestion as I was extremely intent on a career in natural medicine. Still, the concept of writing my thoughts down to possibly help or inspire others always rested in the deep crevices of my mind.

It was not until I faced my own personal health challenge and my subsequent C.U.R.E. that the desire to put my thoughts down on paper was reawakened. At first it was in the form of a blog, but as I began to work this healing process with my own patients I came to the realization that an internet blog was not sufficient.

What I have learned from my own body and through countless patients is not something to be kept behind closed doors or privacy curtains. Instead, it is something that I deeply and profoundly feel must be shared with as many people as possible. In this day and age of big brother watching, I wanted to create a title for this book that would grab people's attention, yet keep me off the radar of those who like to silence the non-traditional thinkers (how am I doing so far?). My heart wanted to shout from the rooftops "I am cured!!!" but the sensible side of me feared the backlash of such a proclamation. However, the word "cure" would not leave me and that is when I decided to turn a word into an acronym.

C.U.R.E.—Cultivating Unlimited Rejuvenating Energy

Cultivate: *To foster the growth of; to develop or improve by education or training; train; to refine*

When I hear the word "cultivate," I think about a backyard garden where a loving person carefully tends to the soil, seeds, and plants, providing them with water, unrestricted sunlight, and protection from too many pests (naturally of course), allowing the plants to do what they were meant to do. To grow, flourish, and thrive so as to one day provide us with their fruit. It is in the support, not artificial manipulation of the plants that allows them to propagate. Our bodies are no different. Supporting the human body with real nutrition in its cleanest form will allow health to propagate unrestricted.

Unlimited: *Unrestricted; unconfined; boundless; infinite; vast*

So too is the body's ability to heal; unlimited in all ways. There is no disease that cannot be healed, though there are people who cannot heal due to timing or unwillingness to try. The ability of our body to heal is only limited by our willingness to put in the effort.

Rejuvenating: *To restore to a former state; make fresh or new again; to make young again; restore to youthful vigor, appearance*

There is no doubt that when you see my before and after photos there is a rejuvenation that has occurred. I am often told that I look younger now than even before I had a thyroid storm! On a daily basis our bodies rejuvenate themselves automatically! Every 120 days our bone marrow creates new red blood cells. Every 49 days new bladder cells are born. New skin and hair cells bloom every 30 days. Even after only five days we have new cells to line our stomach. The human body knows no limits and will strive for life *even* when we abuse it with alcohol, cigarettes, processed food, fat, and salt.

Energy: *The capacity for vigorous activity; available power; an adequate or abundant amount of such power; Qi*

It is with energy, Qi as it is known in traditional Chinese medicine (TCM), that we shine where our bodies move from the darkness of illness to the light of optimal health and wellbeing. Energy is what drives us to do for others and to make the world a greater place. Most Americans move through their lives with a serious energy deficiency. Without this amazing electrical force, cells cannot function, heal, or rejuvenate. And so, we Cultivate Unlimited Rejuvenating Energy allowing the body to cure what ails it.

In my acupuncture practice I have the great pleasure and blessing to participate in this process with countless individuals who suffer from a vast array of illnesses and diseases. The healing of the body is just one benefit of this process. The healing of the mind and spirit are another. Often those who come to heal a physical issue do not realize that their spirit is "sick" as well. That is where we shine!

I am truly blessed to have been given an amazing group of healers to work with and share in our patients' accomplishments. There is no doubt in my mind that the love shown to our patients by the staff at Partners in Healing is a tremendous part of their healing process. These incredible teachers, colleagues, supporters, and friends make up the team at Partners in Healing. They create the "partnership" in this journey to health and I would be lost without them.

I constantly strive to do all I can to C.U.R.E. those who entrust their health to me, but it is and always will be the patient's responsibility to take their health into their own hands, as I had to do with mine. When I met Dr. Robert Morse in 2011, I was greeted with a loving smile and a big bear hug. I knew at that moment I was in the right place; a healing place. But Dr. Morse made it clear that it was my responsibility to create healing in my own body. There were no shortcuts. No magic wands. This was going to take work. His boldness, candor, love, and compassion were the vibrations I needed to cause a miracle in my life.

As I take in a deep cleansing breath and let it out in a soothing sigh, I struggle to find the words worthy of honoring such a spirit as Robert. Without him, this book, nor I, would exist. He saved my life and that of all he touches in both health and spirit. He has taught me how to profoundly help others through educating, understanding, and of course detoxifying them. Robert's respect for those he helps on their healing journey is the key to his success. If not for respect, he would just push through an appointment in eight minutes, never looking up from a file folder of numbers and tests. Instead he takes his time with each new patient, explaining how the body works and why we get sick. In this way, the patient understands and eagerly awaits instructions as to how to get well via detoxification and rejuvenation. It has been my honor to be his patient, his devotee, his student, and his friend. Though he no longer takes on new patients, his sharing of knowledge has taken practitioners like me to places I never thought possible. I have been utterly blessed to have him as my mentor.

As with any endeavor, it truly *"takes a village."* I am blessed to live in a community of people who believe that the human body has an innate ability and desire to heal and be well. If we look to nature, respect and honor the species and spirit that we are, there is no question that we can live a happy, healthy, vibrant and soulful life for many, many years. Enjoy the journey, be good to yourselves and I thank you for taking a few moments out of your life to read this book. It is my deepest wish that the information in this book inspires you, makes you smile, and heals you in both body and soul as it did me.

In health and love,

Rosanne Calabrese AP

> *"You need to spend time crawling alone through shadows to truly appreciate what it is to stand in the sun."*

- Shaun Hick

C | U | R | E *quotes*

chapter one
My Story

The question is always how to begin. I could start at the beginning. At the time, I didn't know when the beginning took place, or even what I was beginning, for that matter. Instead, I'll begin in the middle, because it was in the middle when everything started.

On October 15th, 2010, I woke up for work without an alarm. It wasn't unusual for me to wake on my own; I have woken up without an alarm for many years, even though I always set one just in case. On that particular morning, I awoke at 4:45 a.m., about two hours earlier than usual. My morning routine usually consisted of showering, blow drying my hair, quickly grabbing a piece of fruit, and then running off to my acupuncture office. My routine wasn't always this hectic, mind you. But as the years went by, I found it more and more difficult to find the time to get my paperwork done, in addition to treating all of my patients over the course of an eight hour day. My answer to this problem? Extending my workday on both ends and grabbing something here or there for breakfast and lunch.

As I said before, I awoke that day at 4:45 a.m. I was startled awake by an unusual pounding in my chest and a powerful, constant swishing sound in my ears, like that of my horse swatting flies with his tail. Alarmed and anxious, I sat up in bed and assessed my surroundings. My husband, Anthony, lay next to me sleeping quietly. The room was dark, and it was nowhere near time for me to get up. The dog was snoring lightly, so as far as I could tell, I wasn't roused by any loud noises. I took another quick glance at the clock. "Ok," I thought, "I have almost two hours to get some more sleep," so I laid back down.

As I nestled back under my soft covers, the sound of the movement of the sheets momentarily drowned out the loud swishing in my ears. However, once I got back into a comfortable sleeping position, the pounding started in my chest all over again, and then the swishing in my ears returned, both at a very quick pace. I took a few breaths, shook my head in a gesture of futility, and realized that sleep was no longer on the agenda. I decided to get up and got ready for work.

I worked a full day, arrived home, and had dinner without incident. Later that night, I drifted off to sleep around 11:00 p.m., only to wake at 3:00 a.m. The sound of my heartbeat in my ears had returned with a vengeance.

OK, I knew I had been working a lot over the past... 12 years. Missing yoga classes, always promising myself that I would start meditating, relaxing, or taking a vacation... Tomorrow. What better time than 3:00 a.m. to start doing something beneficial for myself, like meditating? I focused on my breathing, in and out, deep and rhythmic... Yet my heartbeat continued pounding in my ears, 'lub dub, lub dub, lub dub.' The swishing noise became louder and louder. Stronger and stronger in my chest until it felt as if my heart would explode! I was at my wit's end and decided to retreat to the most relaxing place on earth... My rocking chair.

For 14 nights I started out in bed, only to find myself in an absolutely anxious state within 30 minutes. Moving to the living room with my pillow and blanket wrapped around me, I curled up in my rocking chair hoping for some rest. The rhythmic rocking of the chair and squeaking of the wood, as well as my upright position, seemed to drown out the sounds within my head and the beating within my chest. I wasn't able to truly sleep but at least I was more peaceful, all the while wondering why I couldn't calm myself down.

Anxiety stricken, I finally told my husband I needed to find a doctor who could talk me off the ledge, so to speak. I needed a professional to tell me that I had been working too hard the past 12 years as a firefighter and acupuncture student, who became a fire fighting Acupuncture Physician, who was now running her own full time holistic health clinic! I needed someone in a white lab coat to give me permission to take it easy, work less, and take a vacation...but what I got instead turned my life on its head!

I sat on the exam table across from the D.O. (Doctor of Osteopathic Medicine) I had found in the yellow pages, Dr. K. He had the same last name as the orthopedic that treated my pelvic fracture two and a half years prior, so he seemed as good a choice as any. Once in the exam room, I explained how I didn't really know why I was there. I was certain that I would never take an anti-anxiety pill or anything else he'd probably prescribe to calm me down. I told him that I tend to work too much and that my heart rate had been about 100 - 110 BPM for two weeks prior, keeping me from getting any sleep. He looked up from his clipboard, over the top of his crooked glasses and asked, "Do you think it has anything to do with that big goiter on your neck?"

"Goiter?!" I replied. "What goiter? I don't have a goiter!"

"Darling," the doctor replied, "You've got a goiter." He led me to a mirror and palpated my throat in front of it, outlining a huge protruding thickness on my neck. My heart sunk as I desperately tried to come up with a reason for this lump in my throat (both literally and figuratively). The next hour was filled with blood tests, ultrasounds, and tears as I called my husband to inform him that it wasn't stress which was keeping me awake at night - it was much more serious.

Dr. K called the next morning with the test results. I was diagnosed with a hyperthyroid. Since he did not perform an antibody test, he was unable to identify the reason for my overactive thyroid. Was it Graves' disease? Hashimoto's? Thyroiditis? Nodular goiter? What exactly was causing my thyroid to enlarge?

I asked Dr. K what the course of action was. His explanation was as casual as if I were making an appointment to get my legs waxed. "Oh, it's simple. You take a radioactive iodine pill, stay away from pregnant women and children for five days and then, after your thyroid dies, you take the prescription drug Synthroid for the rest of your life."

SIMPLE!? This didn't sound simple to me, it sounded barbaric! Why on earth would I take a pill that causes me to be so toxic and radioactive that I have to stay away from pregnant women and children? Killing off one of my own body parts? It sounded insane!

Was there no other way? I see twenty patients a day in my acupuncture office, and inevitably one or two each week are on Synthroid and still suffer from thyroid symptoms, including weight gain and fatigue. This was not a solution for me and I told Dr. K that I wanted to find another way.

"So what is plan B?" I asked.

"There is no plan B," he told me. "This is your only hope."

"But why did I get this? What caused my hyperthyroidism? If we find the cause, won't we find the cure?"

After all, this is what I have told my patients for the past nine years in my acupuncture practice. If we search for the cause of your illness and find it, then we can reverse (dare I say cure) the illness! This is what every practitioner of natural medicine believes. I decided to leave allopathic medicine behind and search for a natural way to heal my thyroid. But first, I still needed allopathic technology to find out what I was actually trying to heal.

Dr. G was the medical doctor I had met when I was a Miami Dade Fire Fighter for fourteen years prior to becoming an Acupuncture Physician. I contacted Dr. G and was seen immediately. After a two hour conversation, Dr. G sent me to Quest Labs armed with a dozen prescriptions for every blood test known to man! Twenty-one vials of blood were drawn that day and after a few more days Dr. G contacted me with the results. I had over five times the antibodies for Hashimoto's disease and even more antibodies for Graves' disease. My body was on the attack...of itself!

Hashimoto's and Graves' are described by Western medicine as "autoimmune" diseases. In essence, the body is attacking itself for some unknown reason. This is why doctors just look to kill the subject being attacked thus halting the process. But that doesn't really make sense, does it? I mean, if we don't know (or care) why the body has decided to turn on itself, and we kill or remove that part it is attacking, how do we know that this rogue body won't go after another poor unsuspecting gland, tissue or organ in the future? The answer is that we don't know. And, oftentimes, it does start attacking another part of the body! There are many individuals who have fought Graves' disease by killing the thyroid, only to be diagnosed years later with Rheumatoid Arthritis, Multiple Sclerosis or Lupus. So why would I want to just address the symptom and not the cause?

The truth is that Western medicine rarely addresses the cause, unless of course they can spend billions of dollars studying the elusive genome (this is a technique used to distract the public from their role in the disease process and thus their ability to reverse it). Otherwise, it's just cut, radiate, drug, chemo, and move along until the side effects of these processes catch up with the patient and then of course, do it all again! No, not me! I vowed to find another way.

Dr. G seemed to think she had another way, although she was not completely sure. She had a theory that all of the deficiencies in my blood were the cause of my body going rogue. If we could just balance out all of the nutrient abnormalities, then my body could heal. This sounded good although there was no explanation as to *why* I had so many nutritional deficiencies. After all, I prided myself in my extensive knowledge of diet and nutrition.

Dr. G practiced what is known as "functional medicine" which looks at the body as a whole (go figure) and takes into consideration that illness is caused by deficiencies of nutrients as well as genetics. Again, this sounded good to me at the time. Dr. G prescribed a beta blocker to slow down my heart rate (symptom control) and a massive number of supplements as well as a protein powder from Metagenix. She also made some dietary recommendations which included pumpkin seeds and Brazil nuts. I followed everything she prescribed to a T, swallowing dozens of pills a day. But I still felt as if I needed something more.

Stress had played a huge role in my life. I am somewhat of a perfectionist when it comes to taking care of my patients, and all others in my life, for that matter. As I said before, I was a fire fighter with Miami Dade for fourteen years and one of the first female fire fighters in Deerfield Beach before that. I had worked full time while I went to school to earn my Master's degree in acupuncture, then worked both jobs for two years until 2004 when I retired from the fire department to be a full time acupuncture physician. I found myself working longer and longer hours and taking less time off.

While I felt that the plan to use supplements to get rid of my thyroid problem was a good one, it would not help me deal with stress.

The only way to do that, I felt, was to remove myself from some of my stressors, including my beloved acupuncture practice. I've been a long-time fan of Dr. Gabriel Cousens, his book Conscious Eating, and his documentary film Simply Raw. This was all I needed to choose my path of healing…my body, mind, and spirit. I decided to travel to Patagonia, Arizona and experience The Tree of Life Rejuvenation Center firsthand. There I could eat fresh, organic, raw food; get reacquainted with nature, and meditate, meditate, meditate. Although my office manager felt I was taking a "vacation," I knew removing myself from my environment was the only way to completely heal.

I was feeling worse and worse. The beta blockers were not working. I was enduring massive waves of anxiety, night sweats, hot flashes, and even experienced body odor for the first time since becoming vegan. It was now November 2010, nearly four weeks since my symptoms had started, and I was finally on an airplane to Arizona. I arrived in Phoenix to spend the night at my brother and sister-in-laws' house before making the three-hour drive into the desert. When I awoke in my family's guest room the next morning, I felt as if I had caught the flu. My body was hot and achy all over. I was very fatigued and my eyes were swollen. The thought of the three-hour drive alone was completely unappealing, but I knew I had to do it.

Arriving at the Tree of Life that afternoon was a huge relief. The GPS did its job, even though I no longer had a phone signal. The staff was friendly and welcoming as they checked me in, gave me a tour and told me what the next day and a half would be like. That night would be my last meal for 24 hours. The next morning would start the blood and saliva testing to help determine what protocol I would be following. I would also be meeting with the Naturopathic Doctor (ND) after the testing and then be allowed to eat a full meal at dinner. I made my way to my "home" for the next three weeks, unpacked my things, and then carried my laptop to the cafe area where I could grab Wi-Fi and Skype my husband. I was feeling very weary with the lingering flu-like symptoms, but a feeling of calm had come over me knowing that I was in a place with people who spoke my language. These people did not want me to radiate and kill my thyroid any more than I wanted to. They trusted in the healing power of the body and good nutrition. They believed that mother Earth was able to provide all I needed to heal. I was in the right place at the right time and the next three weeks were going to prove all of the medical doctors wrong.

After a nice chat with my husband I went to dinner - a wonderful array of raw dishes from soup to nuts! Both guests and staff were kind, pleasant, and eager to share their stories. After finishing dinner and a huge fresh green vegetable drink, I said my good nights and headed up the hill to my room. It was starkly furnished with no TV, telephone, or turn down service, but I wasn't there for the frills, I was there for the miracles.

I had a restless sleep that night and woke the next morning around 5:00 a.m. I was instructed to skip breakfast so that I could begin testing first thing in the morning. As I drove my rental car down to the clinic at the foot of the hill, I began to feel light-headed. Once in the clinic, the nurse started with a saliva test to be followed with my first fasting blood test. I felt extremely weak, not because I was in the midst of a 24 hour fast, but because the anxiety and jitters would not allow my body to rest. I felt tired and wired at the same time, and I just couldn't get my heart to calm down. After the saliva test and first blood test, I was given an apple and instructed to take fifteen minutes to eat it.

My next blood test would not be for 90 minutes, so I was given a choice of going back to my room or waiting in the patient lounge. My choice seemed obvious. The lounge was just a few steps away and was warmed by a large picture window where the Arizona sun streamed through. I curled up in the corner of a small couch and waited to be called. I was cold and hot at the same time. I thought I was possibly catching a cold or flu, but no sore throat although my voice was becoming quite hoarse. I must have dozed off until the nurse came in to bring me back for the next blood test.

I became increasingly nauseated as she drew my blood and then handed me a large glass of water with spirulina. I was instructed to drink the entire glass and return in an hour for my next blood test. If I thought I was nauseous before, the deep green of the spirulina really put me over the edge. But I didn't lose my cookies. I kept it all down! Again, I returned to lie on the sofa, feeling worse and worse as if my body were unable to move. Several more times, the nurse returned and several more blood draws were made. I was finally done around 2:00 p.m. and was encouraged to go to the dining area for lunch. I was not really hungry and just grabbed some fruit and returned to my room. I had an appointment at 4:00 p.m. to see the naturopath so I thought I would rest until then. But I was unable to completely rest. My heartbeat was swishing in my ears again. I took a beta blocker and watched the clock, waiting for something to change.

At 3:45 I drove down the hill to the clinic and returned to the couch, curling up in the corner. By 4:00 the naturopathic doctor walked in and escorted me to her office. I found myself in a cozy, warm office with Native American arts and crafts all around. The doctor was caring and concerned, asking everything from what was going on with my health to what I did for a living. She wanted to know about my work hours as well as my play time. She asked about stress, how I lived my life, my work ethic, and my relationships. This was not a typical doctor visit, this was more like how I treated my own patients. I found myself breaking down in tears, unable to control my emotions. I thought it was because I finally had a medical professional listening to me instead of me listening to others. As we spoke, my heart pounded stronger and stronger in my chest and ears. It was an emotional time. What I didn't know was that it was the start of something very, very bad.

After the doctor calmed me down, we discussed the program and how I could get my body back to optimal health. Step number one: Joining her and the other guests in the temple for the evening meditation. I went back to my room, showered and changed clothes (I had become very hot and sweaty during the testing process and consultation) and drove halfway down the hill to the temple.

The temple was a round adobe style building with a peaked roof and wooden door. As I walked up the gravel walkway and approached the door I noticed several pairs of flip flops, shoes, and sneakers outside. I slid off my sandals and added them to the pile, and then walked inside. The single room temple was dimly lit and I let my eyes adjust before I found a place to sit. The shoeless participants sat on pillows around the fire pit in the center of the room. As my eyes focused, one of the staff began to chant and the meditation began. The room was quiet except for the crackle of the fire and my heart pounding in my chest and ears. The chants of 'om' continued. As the room seemed to get warmer and warmer, I became more and more uncomfortable and agitated by my pounding heart and increasing body heat. Everyone sat still and quiet as I squirmed in my seat trying to get comfortable, trying not to panic. But the panic became stronger and stronger and when I finally couldn't take it anymore and was about to stand up, the chimes were rung and the meditation was over.

I was the first one out of the temple and in my car. Dinner was about to be served in the cantina, but all I could think about was getting something cold to drink. I don't drink soda, but the fever that was growing inside my body, along with the nausea, had me craving a tall icy glass of ginger ale. Unfortunately, all I could get from the cantina was a green vegetable juice. I took the juice in a "to-go" cup and went back to my room. I had filled the shelf alongside my bed with supplements that Dr. G had recommended as well as my prescription of beta blockers. I sat down on the edge of my bed with my green juice and began swallowing pills, hoping to calm my body down. But as the minutes ticked by, my symptoms became worse. I was incredibly agitated and panicked; my whole body was shaking uncontrollably. In an attempt to triage myself, I took out my cell phone, opened up the stop watch application, placed my fingers on the pounding pulse in my neck and started to count. After 60 seconds, my heart rate was 132 just sitting there! I was sweating profusely now and no matter how much I drank I was still thirsty and had cotton mouth. I needed help but there was no one around. Looking out my front door I could see that the other rooms were dark so I assumed that everyone was still having dinner down the hillside in the cantina. There were no phones in the rooms and my cell phone had no signal in the hills of Arizona. The only call I could make was to 9-1-1.

I dialed. For a moment I felt better, or at least at ease. There was a voice on the other end who said that they could help. All I had to do was "sit tight." When the volunteer rescue crew arrived they took out the EKG and pulse oximeter and confirmed that my heart rate was now 142. My body temperature was 103 and blood pressure was climbing as high as 130/84 which was very high for me. I was in a thyroid storm. The volunteer crew advised the county rescue crew by radio what they had and that the incoming crew would have to transport me to St. Joseph's Hospital in Tucson, nearly 90 minutes away.

The county crew wasted no time starting an IV and putting me in the back of the rescue truck. 45 minutes into the ride I was finally able to get a cell phone signal and called my husband in Florida. It was midnight at home and he was sleeping. When he answered the phone, I wanted to be sure not to scare him, so the first words out of my mouth were "Everything is alright, but I am on my way to the hospital." We spoke for a few minutes as he gathered information about my condition and the hospital that we were headed to and promised to fly out to Tucson first thing in the morning. I hung up the phone telling him not to worry, all while I was in a full on panic!

The next six days were the most treacherous days of my life. I had been in the hospital once before for four days due to a pelvic fracture and all I could say, is I would take 10 pelvic fractures over a thyroid storm any day. It took two different thyroid medications, beta blockers, steroids, ibuprofen, two hospitals and six days to calm the storm enough to allow me to go home. I had lost 11 pounds in six days, my skin was dry, my hair was brittle and falling out and although I had lost a significant amount of weight (I was only 118lbs before the thyroid storm) my face was extremely swollen with severe edema around my eyes. I was so incredibly weak that my husband had to get a wheelchair to transport me to and from the airplane. I was now on 30mg of Methimazol each day. This powerful drug artificially subdued my symptoms, but at a price. The hope was that the end of the thyroid storm would be the end of my problems, but that is not how the thyroid and Graves' disease works.

Upon arriving home I went from the airport directly to my Acupuncture Physician's office, Dr. F. He prepared an herbal formula that would help to calm down my thyroid and all of the "internal heat" that was burning up my "yin." This process was far more natural than Western medicine and followed traditional

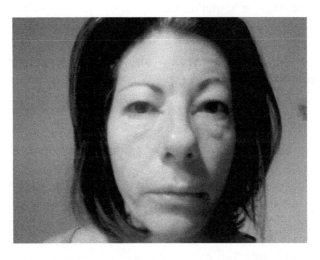

Approximately 2 weeks following the thyroid storm

Chinese medicine principles. I remained on the medication that the hospital gave me and trusted that the herbs would not interfere with the Methimazol that the doctor prescribed. Dr. F said that my thyroid would soon burn out from constant hyperactivity and become hypo-thyroidal, which concerned me. I wanted my thyroid to function normally, not too fast or too slow. Anthony took me home and ran out to pick up dinner. Soon after, I went to bed hoping that the next day would be better.

Although my thyroid storm was "under control," my symptoms were not gone. That first night at home was not much better than the nights before I had traveled to The Tree of Life. I was awoken at around one in the morning by sweating and a rapid heartbeat. It was only 90 beats per minute but it terrified me. I went to the living room and tried to sleep on the sofa. By 6:30 that morning I had had enough and slipped out of the house to the Cleveland Clinic's emergency room. They followed the usual procedures and drew my blood only to find my thyroid numbers through the roof (which was no surprise). They wanted to admit me, but I had been there and done that and I wasn't going to lie in a hospital bed again. I got on the phone from the ER and called the Cleveland Clinic appointment line. I wished I had this much luck when buying a lotto ticket….there was a cancelation for the 4pm appointment and I actually got in! Maybe my luck was turning around!

Cleveland Clinic has a reputation for being on the cutting edge of medical technology. This was my chance to see a doctor who was not the same old cookie cutter prescription writer. I was excited to meet this man.

As Anthony and I sat in the exam room, I felt hopeful that Dr. D would give us the good news that we were looking for…that there were other options to radiating my thyroid. He entered the room in a long white lab coat and clipboard under his arm with a kind smile. He extended his hand to me and Anthony, and then sat down in the desk chair and opened my file. He had copies of that morning's blood work and copies of previous tests that I had given to the nurse. He then proceeded to explain that my thyroid was working overtime and that the dose of Methimazole that I was on was appropriate. He advised me to use the beta blockers to slow my heart rate so that I would be comfortable. Periodic blood tests would also enable him to reduce my Methimazole accordingly until I could be taken off of it, probably in about 18 months. Then, the clincher… Once off the medication for seven days, he could then proceed to radiate my thyroid. "Holy crap! Are we here again," I thought?

"But Dr. D…Isn't there another way?" I begged. Sadly, the answer was no. While there are some rare occasions when patients' symptoms will go away permanently following an 18 month course of Methimazole, there was no indication, based on my lab tests, that I would be one of those patients. This was a significant and serious case of Grave's Disease.

I returned home upset, scared, and extremely disappointed. I thought Cleveland Clinic was the best in the business. I thought they had new and innovative ways to treat illness rather than the antiquated search and destroy method. I plopped down on the sofa and laid there for the next four weeks.

I was down but not out. In those four weeks, between visits from friends and family, I began to do my own research. Amazon is an amazing resource to obtain books, both physical and digital versions.

I purchased every book I could find on the thyroid, hyperthyroidism, Graves' disease, and natural medicine. I referenced and cross referenced through the internet using every search engine I could find. I ordered supplements through my office, purchased them at the health food stores, and resumed seeing Dr. F and Dr. G. Each day was a whirlwind of appointments. There was always some kind of appointment, whether it was for acupuncture, herbs, cranial sacral therapy, chiropractic, blood tests, or MD appointments—even in a greatly weakened state, I was on the go, trying to get better and keep my thyroid. Even though I had been vegan for 18 years, someone convinced me that I needed more protein, so I even began eating eggs!

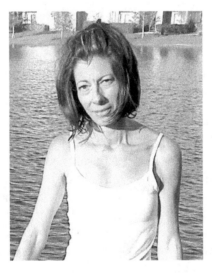

Just prior to starting detox

But nothing was working. My eyes continued to swell, I still had bouts of rapid heartbeat, I was weak, skinny, and my goiter continued to grow! The drug allowed me to function, albeit at a slow pace, but the thyroid problem itself did not retreat. Blood tests showed the thyroid suppressive quality of Methimazole, but I was not healing my body. I returned to work in the beginning of December for only two days a week. I felt like a hypocrite and a failure. Why would anyone want to see me for medical advice when

I could not even cure myself? Yes, I knew it was a lot to expect me to "cure" Graves' disease, but I still thought if I was worth my weight as a natural medicine physician, I should be able to handle it.

I was feeling stronger when an old patient of mine invited me to lunch. It had been a while since I socialized, and I thought lunch out sounded like a good idea. Little did I know, it ended up being the greatest idea of my life!

Francesca was a patient that originally came to me with some digestive issues. She improved with acupuncture, herbs, and homeopathy. Years later she returned with a severe and acute onset of rheumatoid arthritis. She was deathly afraid of going on the chemotherapy drug Methotrexate (with good reason) which is standard protocol for RA, and wanted to conquer this horrible disease naturally. So she came back to my office for some help. I had her make serious nutritional changes—become vegan, attend weekly acupuncture treatments, visit an infrared sauna, and begin a regimen of herbs and homeopathic injections. Within six months her blood work was normal.

One day in mid-February 2011, Francesca and I decided to have lunch at the Greenwave Café, a small local raw food school and restaurant. When you are in the natural medicine world, the circle is tight and everyone knows everyone. Raoul was a Dade County Fire Fighter 15 years before I was. He left for personal reasons several years before I got hired, including his health. I left to help others as an acupuncture physician. Raoul and I met soon after he and his wife opened the Greenwave Café. It was the obvious choice of a lunch location for Francesca and me.

As we sat down at the counter to order our lunch, Raoul walked in the front door. Like a local celebrity, everyone wanted to say hello to Raoul as he walked past. They clamored to ask him health and dietary questions, hoping that he would impart words of wisdom, hope, and inspiration. Raoul had reversed high blood pressure, excess weight, and prostate cancer with raw food and thus had his finger on the pulse of the raw food and natural health movement. When he finally made it behind the counter, Francesca and I were eating our salad. Raoul took a double take and realized it was me sitting opposite him. His expression quickly went from a broad, toothy smile to a somber gaze. He reached forward, clasped my hands, and said "Rosanne, I heard you were ill. Tell me what is going on." I explained the whole story while he listened intently. Finally, when I was finished, he reached under the counter, pulled out a brochure and said, "You have to call this man...NOW!" I finished lunch, got back in my car, and made the call.

The first opening that Dr. Morse had was two months away (March 2011). I had already scheduled several phone consultations with natural medicine "experts" in Arizona and California, as well as an in-office appointment in Michigan at the beginning of May. I was not letting anything stand in my way of getting better and keeping my thyroid, but call after call left me more melancholy and disappointed than before.

The night before I was to drive three hours to see Dr. Morse, I consulted with a doctor in California for 50 minutes. After giving his secretary my credit card number and authorizing a $250 charge, I was told that I was the most complicated case of Graves' disease and Hashimoto's that he had seen. He advised that there were protocols that I could research on my own which used the medication that I was already on, but in a different way.

I was millimeters away from cancelling my appointment with Dr. Morse the next day. I felt hopeless and weak. I was losing the fight in me. The fight that had drove me at the age of 26 and only 113lbs to become a firefighter; the fight that drove me to leave the fire department after 15 years of service and strike out on my own to become an Acupuncture Physician...

The fight in me was fading.

The next morning, my husband and I got dressed and headed out for our three hour ride to the west coast of Florida. When we arrived we were greeted by a friendly staff in an informal and relaxed setting. They were extremely organized, handing me paperwork and a three ring binder to read while others packaged bottles of herbs for shipment to who-knows-where. Their smiles were authentic and made me feel safe. They offered us a raw food snack bar and asked us to have a seat.

Moments later we were escorted into a large office lined with bookshelves filled with hundreds of books (many of which I had in my library!) and a large unusual desk adorned in colorful plastic fruit! Behind the desk stood a white haired man whose hair and smile reminded me of Colonel Sanders. He extended his hand to me, then Anthony, and offered us a seat. "So nice to meet you," he said as he flipped through my medical history form. "So what brings you to the West Coast?" he asked. As I went through my story, he listened intently until I was completely finished. It was hard to hold back the tears after detailing months of suffering with rapid heartbeat, hot flashes, swelling of my eyes, and enormous amounts of anxiety and irritability followed by disappointment after disappointment.

"I understand," Dr. Morse said. "This has been a hard time for you." As he flipped through the medical history forms I had filled out, I noticed him shaking his head. I braced myself for more bad news.

"Is this it?" He asked.

"Yes," I replied in a shaky voice.

"This is all that is going on?" He asked again.

"I HAVE GRAVES' DISEASE"! I blurted in a somewhat aggravated tone. For God's sake, did he not listen to my pain and suffering? This was A BIG DEAL!

"Oh, that's easy then," he replied with a huge white smile.

"Easy? How is this easy when every specialist from California to Arizona to the University of Miami to Cleveland Clinic is telling me that it is EXTREMELY complicated?" I asked.

"Well my dear, I know you are an Acupuncture Physician, but would you mind terribly if I tell you how the body works?" Dr. Morse asked in his kind southern drawl.

"Sure," I replied and sat back to listen to his profound, yet simplistic explanation of how the body works, how I got sick, and how I could recover and keep my thyroid.

Dr. Morse explained how the lymphatic system is the key to optimal function of all cells and how an alkaline diet along with the right herbs is the only way to get the body functioning the way God and nature intended! He explained how the body can never be balanced by using isolates (isolated nutrients such as vitamins and minerals), and that if you suffer from malabsorption (which most of us do) then the body is not absorbing all of the pills you are taking anyway. By the end of the consultation, my husband was asking if he could participate in the "program" along with me.

"Of course you can," Dr. Morse replied with an air of excitement!

Dr. Morse took a photograph of my eyes (an iridology procedure) and then Anthony's. He briefly described what he saw and how that impacted his decision of what herbs to prescribe for each of us. He explained how diet is the key to the success of the detoxification and rejuvenation program and asked us to commit to 12 weeks. We did not hesitate. This was the first and only doctor to give me hope to keep my thyroid and reverse this illness and I grabbed on to it like a life boat on the Titanic!

I loved what this doctor was saying. It resonated with everything I believe in and what I share with my patients. Suddenly I forgot about my illness and began thinking of my patients and all of the people I could help. I wanted to learn more about what Dr. Morse did and how I could do the same thing with my patients. As luck would have it, Dr. Morse would be teaching a 40 hour class approximately one month after my visit with him. There was no doubt where I was going to be in a month…In Dr. Morse's class, in the front row!

Once back home, Anthony and I went to the local health food grocery store and stocked up on lots of fresh organic fruit and vegetables. The next morning our day began with fresh fruit smoothies filled with oranges, pineapple, berries and mango…Mmmmm! Next we mixed our liquid herbs into some of the smoothie and drank them down followed by some herbal capsules. Later in the day I brewed some special herbal tea. Snacks consisted of fresh fruit or vegetable juices. Lunch and dinner were either fruit or vegetable salads, or steamed vegetables with avocado or sweet potato. It was simple, healthy, and hearty. There were no limitations on the amount of food I could eat and I found that I was rarely hungry. Suddenly my energy levels began to increase, and deep down, I knew I was on the right track (although there was still an element of fear in my mind).

One week into the cleanse I had a scheduled appointment with my endocrinologist. I had made a conscious decision not share anything with him about the program I was on. After all, I was only seven days into it, and although I had a crazy notion that my thyroid was already shrinking, I did not want to make a fool of myself and tell him I had the cure for Graves' disease. Dr. D asked me the usual questions, looked at my blood work and then stood up to examine and palpate my thyroid. As he stood next to me and placed his fingers on my throat, I held my breath. His fingers moved across the skin that covered my thyroid slowly and then faster, back and forth. Finally Dr. D stopped, stepped back, looked at me and said, "Well, it seems your thyroid is smaller."

"Are you sure?" I asked, with a slight grin on my face.

"Yes, I am sure," he replied. "I examine your thyroid every three or four weeks and have only seen it grow larger. I definitely can tell when it is shrinking."

I left it alone. Again, I did not want to get my hopes up, only to be disappointed down the road. But the news that my thyroid was smaller was BIG! My thyroid had continued to grow even while taking the Methimazole. Now, just one week into the detoxification it was already smaller. Dr. D asked me to lower my dose of Methimazole and make an appointment in four weeks. I left his office with serenity and a smile.

As the weeks went on, detoxification symptoms crept in. The skin on my face was breaking out with acne and strange, itchy red welts appeared on my legs. I was extremely tired at times, and suffered from nausea, headaches, and body aches. Dr. Morse explained that detox symptoms would appear as I moved deeper into the process. He also said that old injuries could start hurting again and symptoms of past illness could return, alongside new aches, pains and discomforts. All of this was due to the body clearing out its lymphatic system, organs, and tissues. My body was spring cleaning! I added another day to my work schedule which put me up to three days a week. I started to visit my horse more often at the barn and although not myself yet, I felt I was definitely on my way. I constantly felt my neck and looked in the mirror. The goiter was becoming visibly smaller now almost by the day! Four weeks went by and I was due to see Dr. D, my endocrinologist, when his office called to reschedule my appointment. They said I would have to wait 11 more weeks before I could see my doctor! That would be a total of 15 weeks since my last appointment and 16 weeks since I began the detoxification. How was I supposed to know if my thyroid was actually smaller?

Well, there were always blood tests. Dr. D gave me several prescriptions for thyroid panels.

Over the next 11 weeks I took about four blood tests. As Dr. D received the results I would get a phone call or email instructing me to lower my medication dosage. Since I had attended Dr. Morse's extensive 40 hour training I was now not only choosing my own herbs for continued detoxification; I was also beginning to treat my patients with this wonderful herbal program and remarkable nutritional plan. Every day was an amazing healing journey and I finally felt blessed to have this thyroid disease! I purchased an iridology camera which gave me an even more profound look into my patients' bodies. As much as I love acupuncture, I felt that I was given a new tool to treat patients more effectively than ever before.

I was pushing through every day both physically and emotionally. There were days that some symptoms would creep in, like rapid heart rate or insomnia, and I would fear the return of a thyroid storm. But then the symptoms would subside and progress would be made.

Finally, week 16 of my detoxification arrived, along with my appointment to the endocrinologist. I had now been off of Methimazole for three weeks and had taken a blood test the day before my appointment. As I walked into Cleveland Clinic alone that day, I was feeling overwhelmed and humbled. All of these doctors, nurses, and scientists spend years of their lives studying and practicing chemical based medicine. I thought to myself, "Who am I to think I can compete with their knowledge and ability?" Suddenly, I doubted my progress. Why? I am not sure. Maybe it was fear; maybe it was the desire to not be arrogant or too sure of myself.

After all, I have a very complicated case according to top doctors in their respective fields. My heart began to race and I wondered if it was my thyroid. When Dr. D's nurse stepped through the waiting room door and called my name, a feeling of calm came over me. Dr. D's nurse had seen me every time I came to Cleveland Clinic. He was a big, body builder type with a teddy bear personality. He gave me a big hug and told me I was looking really good. We walked to the exam room and he took my vitals. "Everything looks good," he said. We chatted a bit until Dr. D walked in.

Dr. D is from South America. He is a very serious man with a kindness about him. As with most doctors, he is often stoic and hard to read. As the nurse stepped out of the room, Dr. D looked at me over the top of his reading glasses and asked "You are off of Methimazole?"

"Yes," I responded with a slightly shaky voice, "for the past 3 weeks."

"Your blood tests are normal!" he said with a very large grin, "What did you do?"

A huge sigh of relief came from my chest. "Oh doc, you don't want to know the answer to that!"

"Actually, I do," he replied.

For the next few minutes I told Dr. D everything I had done over the past 16 weeks, from herbs (which I brought some sample bottles of) to my diet. He didn't say a word, he just listened. Then he stood up and asked permission to palpate my thyroid. It was practically normal! Only a slight discrepancy from left to right (the left side was always bigger). He stepped back with a look of amazement on his face. Then he caught himself and drew his smile into a more serious expression.

"Well..." he started; "You know what you did is not considered scientific medicine. It has not been part of a double-blind, placebo controlled study.

"Doc," I replied, "I know the herbs and organic fruit and vegetables I ate were not part of a double blind study, but I have a question for you.

Did you want me to get well?"

"Of course I did," he replied.

"So did I," but I wasn't finished. "Did you want to radiate my thyroid?"

"Yes," Dr. D confirmed.

"I didn't," I asserted.

"Do you have to radiate my thyroid?" A rhetorical question, but one I felt it necessary to ask.

"No," he said with a smile.

"Then let's just say the Methimazole fixed my thyroid and call it a day." I was hoping that we could part as friends.

"Rosanne," he said, "I cannot say that the food you ate or the herbs you took helped your thyroid. But, I *can* tell you two things. First, Methimazole is not a curative drug. Second, your case was so severe that I never thought you would go into remission long enough to radiate your thyroid without hospitalization."

I held my hand up and prompted him for a high five!

"Doc," I said, "I believe that what we should take away from this experience is teamwork. I would not be alive today if it were not for emergency medicine and the ability of drugs to get my symptoms under control. That is what allowed me time to use herbs, food, and detoxification to help my body heal. For your part in the process, I thank you."

It came from my heart and it was true. Ignoring all of my symptoms that led up to the thyroid storm caused me to rely upon Western medicine to pull me from the throes of tachycardia and all of the things that went along with a thyroid storm. In hindsight, had I paid attention to the symptoms that spanned a year before the thyroid storm occurred, I may have been able to use acupuncture and natural medicine to correct and avoid such a horrific situation and debilitating disease. But the truth is I didn't pay attention. For all the analyzing and detective work I do for my patients; for all the health education and nutritional advice; for all of the chemical-free products I use to replace their toxic counterparts in the home and work place; for all of the advice I give my patients (especially women in their 30's and 40's) on pacing themselves and lowering their stress levels, I ignored practically everything I stood for. It was for good reason, or so I thought. I was (and continue to be) extremely dedicated to my patients, each and every one of them. But the time came when I finally realized that if self-care is not my number one priority, I cannot be useful to anyone in my life.

Following those 16 weeks of detoxification, I made the decision to continue the process for a full year. It was not difficult, in fact, it was actually quite easy. When I looked at my choices: Killing my thyroid and taking a synthetic drug for the rest of my life; or eating fruit and vegetables and taking amazing herbs created by God and nature and keeping my thyroid, well, the choice was easy.

So today, over five years after beginning the detoxification process, I am happy and healthy…truly! My thyroid levels are normal and I am not on medication. As a matter of fact, even my Graves' antibody level is COMPLETELY NORMAL! Something I was told could never happen. I continue to eat a very clean diet of fruit and vegetables with some sweet potato and occasional brown rice, seeds, and nuts and I delve back into detoxification with a fully alkaline diet and herbs once or twice a year.

What also became very clear to me was the purpose in getting Graves' disease. Yes, I said purpose. I think we can all agree that the most cliché saying in the world is "Everything happens for a reason." How many times have you heard that phrase when you have just broken up with the person you thought you were going to spend the rest of your life, after losing your job, or your beloved pet's death and thought about how much you wanted to slap the person that uttered those words to you? Well, I am one of those people who always said "Everything happens for a reason…" Until my thyroid storm. I have to say, I wanted absolutely no part of this disease or its lessons. The anxiety, hospital stay, weight loss, numerous doctor visits and all the other physical issues that go along with it, made me very reluctant to believe there was a purpose in any of it. But once I began to heal and understand that the body never, ever does anything wrong (and if we do right by it, we can prevent illness and heal disease), I realized that there was an amazing purpose in my illness and subsequent cure.

Today I can boast that I have trained extensively with my healer and mentor Dr. Morse! I continue to practice acupuncture, iridology, and nutritional therapy. I prescribe Chinese and Western herbs and have three massage therapists, two acupuncture physicians, a chiropractor, a yoga therapist and another detox specialist in my office so that I can help my patients in the most appropriate way for their body, mind, and soul. But I must say, the most incredible, natural and effective way in which I can help my patients is by using the detoxification and rejuvenation process that I used myself to cure an incurable disease. I see patients who struggle with obesity, high blood pressure, multiple sclerosis, infertility, cancer, autoimmune disorders, and many other ailments and they all benefit greatly from this process. I continue to treat patients, educate families and lecture the community on how to reverse disease and heal the body, and I feel blessed each and every day that I am able to do it.

14 years ago, when I was getting ready to open my acupuncture practice, I wanted to create three or four names to choose from. But the only name that kept coming into my brain was *Partners in Healing,* because I believe that my practice is about a partnership between the patient and the practitioner. Today as I write this story, the only title that keeps coming to mind is *C.U.R.E. by Cultivating Unlimited Rejuvenating Energy* because that is exactly what this story is about. Our innate ability to truly heal our body, mind and spirit!

Peace, blessings, and true health to all of you!

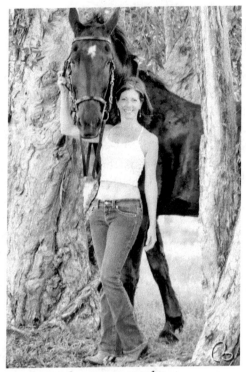

2 years post detox

"We don't get 'struck' with disease. It is not a lightning bolt from the sky! There is a process to disease and a process to reverse it."

- Rosanne Calabrese

C|U|R|E *quotes*

chapter two
The Science of Sickness

Doctors spend countless hours and at least 10 years learning how the body works, and yet when you or I ask, "How did I get Graves' disease?" or "Where did my uncle's cancer come from?" their answer consistently follows this basic premise... "We really don't know what caused your health issue, but we are prepared to treat you." To that statement, I have four questions...

1. If you don't know what caused my illness, should *you* really be the one treating it?

2. Should I accept the treatment of my ailment if doctors and scientists do not understand how it originated?

3. Is the "treatment" for my ailment a cure or is it an ongoing medical process laced with medication, surgery, and/or other toxic therapies?

4. What the heck were you learning in school all of those years if you don't know where my ailment came from or how to cure it?

These questions established the premise that led me to seek natural therapies in an effort to keep my thyroid and reverse Graves' disease. What I discovered during that process is what I will share with you here. *Warning: the information you are about to read may lead to amazing levels of health and wellness as well as healing knowledge that far surpasses your doctor's.* In order to heal the body, you must first understand how it works. This sounds obvious, yet so many highly educated individuals ignore this basic understanding. They delve into science and chemistry so deeply that they cannot see the forest for the trees. The truth (as I have been taught by my healer, mentor, and friend Dr. Robert Morse N.D. as well as discovered through my own healing experience) lies in simplicity. To see the body in its simplicity allows us to support healing in a much more natural and straightforward way.

To understand how our body works, we must first have a grasp of the components which comprise the physical structure of the human body. Of that physical structure, there are three fundamental parts:

1. **Cells**: According to Merriam Webster's dictionary: A small, usually microscopic mass of protoplasm bounded externally by a semipermeable membrane, usually including one or more nuclei and various nonliving products, capable alone or interacting with other cells of performing all the fundamental functions of life, and forming the smallest structural unit of living matter capable of functioning independently.

2. **Blood:** Blood is comprised of plasma and cells that carry oxygen and nutrients to every cell of the body. Blood runs through blood vessels known as arteries and veins. For our purposes we will call the blood the "kitchen" of the body because it provides nutrients or food to every single cell.

3. **Lymph (lymphatic fluid)**: The word *lymph* is derived from the name of the Roman deity of fresh water, Lympha. Lymph is a semi-clear fluid that surrounds every cell of the human body before flowing into its own set of vessels called lymphatic vessels. The lymph fluid makes up nearly two-thirds of all of the fluid of the human body and is responsible for carrying cellular waste away from the cells for processing and elimination from the body. For our purposes, we will call the lymph and lymphatic system the "sewer" of the body.

So now you know the three main components that make up the human body. If you are studying anatomy, you can consider yourself a graduate of anatomy 101!

Once you understand the three main components of the human body, it is time to understand how your cells, blood and lymph play the ultimate role in health and wellness, illness and disease, and finally, in the healing of the body.

Each and every type of cell in the human body has a unique job and function. For example, brain cells have numerous functions unique to them which are vastly different from the functions of skin cells, which are vastly different from the functions of bone cells, and so on. It is not the intention of this book to discuss the function of each cell and tissue. More importantly, I would like to discuss two factors that these seemingly different cells have in common, and how that relates to disease and healing.

1. One thing which each and every cell of the human body has in common—they all have to eat! That is, each cell must take in nutrition (in the form of vitamins, minerals, sugar, and amino acids) in order to carry out its function. No matter what the cell's job, it must take in energy (sugar) and a plethora of other micronutrients (specific to that cell's needs) so that it can stay alive and perform its duties. The way in which the cell is nourished is via the blood, which I referred to earlier as the "kitchen."

   It is the "kitchen" which provides life-giving nutrients to every cell of the body and therefore is the first of the two important points that the cells have in common. Without a blood supply to deliver nutrition to the cells, the cells would starve and rapidly die.

2. After the cells receive nutrition from the blood supply, they carry out their specific metabolic functions and in that process, cellular waste is produced. This metabolic waste must be eliminated from the cell. In other words, the same holds true for the person as for the individual cells. Humans eat and humans poop, cells eat and cells poop! Now this may seem like a strange question, but I have to ask you, how often do you poop in your kitchen? Hopefully your answer is NEVER! Cells do not eliminate waste (with the exception of

CO_2) in their kitchen either! Instead, the cells eliminate their waste into the interstitial space (the space between the cells) which is filled with lymphatic fluid (the sewer system of the body).

The picture below is a great representation of cells and lymph. The fish in the bowl symbolize your cells. They could be brain cells, thyroid cells, liver cells, or prostate cells. You get the picture. Consequently, the water in which they are suspended in represents the lymph. When the fish eliminate waste, it is deposited into the water. When cells eliminate waste, it is deposited into the lymph.

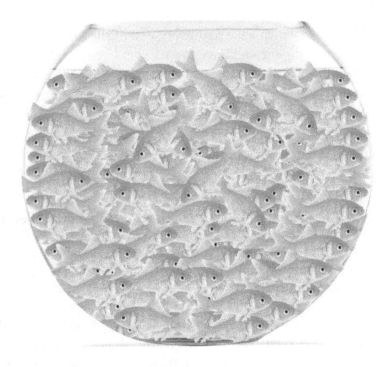

As you can imagine, cellular waste is not meant to linger in this interstitial space. Similar to the flow of water in a river, lymph moves constantly, thus allowing debris to continually be transported away from cells while clean lymph flows in to surround the cells a gain. This lymphatic fluid carries the waste from the interstitial space between the cells into lymphatic vessels (see diagram on next page).

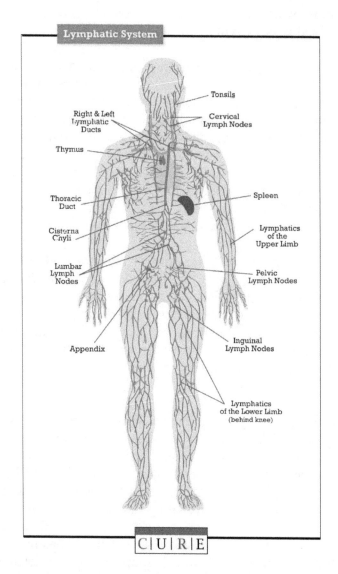

Lymphatic System

Tonsils

Right & Left Lymphatic Ducts

Cervical Lymph Nodes

Thymus

Thoracic Duct

Spleen

Cisterna Chyli

Lymphatics of the Upper Limb

Lumbar Lymph Nodes

Pelvic Lymph Nodes

Appendix

Inguinal Lymph Nodes

Lymphatics of the Lower Limb (behind knee)

C|U|R|E

Lymphatic vessels are the sewer pipes of the body, transporting cellular waste to the vast number of built-in "septic tanks" known as lymph nodes. Lymph nodes are filled with bacteria and white blood cells that serve to further break down cellular waste so that it can ultimately be transported out of the body (we will discuss this shortly).

Lymphatic vessels are in some ways similar to blood vessels in that they are tubes which transport fluid throughout the body. But unlike blood in blood vessels, lymph does not have a "pump" like the heart.

In the circulatory system, the heart pumps blood to the lungs and then throughout the rest of the body, finally returning it to the heart again. There is no such pump in the lymphatic system. Instead, lymph fluid relies upon the contraction and relaxation of surrounding skeletal muscles to push the fluid from the interstitial space into the lymphatic vessels and through the lymphatic system. Once the waste is within the lymphatic vessels, it is processed by the many bacteria and white blood cells found in the lymph nodes so that it can be easily eliminated out of the body via the kidneys (urination), colon (defecation/bowel movements), and skin (sweat).

In very basic and simple terms, this is how the cells of the body function each and every day. Nutrition and energy is delivered via the blood, cellular metabolism occurs, and waste is created and then eliminated into the lymphatic system where it is processed and then finally excreted from the body via the kidneys, colon, and skin. This sounds like a pretty good design, doesn't it? Whether you believe in God or you believe in nature you cannot deny that someone or something got it right!

Yet, if the design is so perfect, one might be compelled to ask, "How do we get sick? Where do illness, disease, tumors, or cell failure come from?" These are excellent questions and some of the pillars of this book. You see, if we can answer the question, "Where does illness come from?" we can then understand how to reverse it and thus Cultivate Unlimited Rejuvenating Energy (C.U.R.E)!

The answer to the question, "How do we get sick?" lies in chemistry. Our body is a massive chemical soup with more elements of chemistry than we have time or intention to discuss here. Therefore, to keep things simple and straightforward, we are going to outline some basic tenets of science. According to science, whether it be in our environment, a chemistry lab, or in our bodies, chemistry is divided into just two sides:
- Acidic chemistry

- Base or alkaline chemistry

Since the human species is an alkaline species (this will be addressed in greater detail in Chapter 7: *Duh*), it stands to reason that the more acidic chemistry we expose the body to via absorption through the skin, respiration and ingestion, the more acidic cellular waste will be produced. The more acidic waste that is produced, the more stress that is placed on the kidneys, colon, and skin. Over time, it becomes more difficult for the body to eliminate waste and thus this waste begins to back up, causing congestion within the interstitial space (between cells). As this acidic congestion lingers around the cells, the cells will become inflamed. Over time, the inflammatory process worsens and affects more and more cells, eventually leading to cellular degeneration. This means that the cells of organs, tissues and glands begin to break down and slowly fail. In other words, if connective tissue becomes inflamed, degenerates and begins to fail, the result would be moderate to severe joint stiffness or pain and decreased ability of the joint to function—for example, difficulty opening a jar, getting dressed, or walking up stairs would be seen. If cells of one of the endocrine glands, known as the thyroid, become inflamed, degenerate and begin to fail, symptoms could include the feeling of sluggishness, lowered body temperature, hair loss, or weight gain. Perhaps if brain cells become congested, inflamed and begin to degenerate, one might forget where they left their keys or call their spouse by the wrong name or struggle to balance a checkbook. All of these "symptoms" of inflammation and cellular degeneration can go on for quite some time, yet all blood tests, CAT scans and other diagnostic tests register as "normal." What is even worse, is the person experiencing these symptoms usually chalks it up to…AGE! Yes, the dreaded cause of disease, getting older! Why, I have had patients in my office who are convinced that their lack of energy, low sex drive, fading memory, body aches, or weight gain were all due to "getting older!" Worse yet, the people who self-diagnosed age as a causative factor were between the ages of 35 and 40! As you can imagine, I vehemently disagreed!

As cellular degeneration continues, eventually enough cells of a particular organ, tissue, or gland will be affected and a disease will be created. Significant symptoms will almost always appear *after* acid buildup in the body, followed by congestion of the lymphatic system, inflammation of cells, tissues organs and glands, degeneration and finally disease! Subsequent to this lengthy process (which exacerbates over tens of years), more serious symptoms will appear. That's right! That is how long illness and the disease process is brewing in the body! Cancer does not appear overnight. It takes five, 10, even 20 years, before a tumor is found or the symptoms of cancer occur. It is the same way with all diseases! You don't go to bed healthy and wake up with Graves' disease, fibromyalgia, or lupus. These conditions take many, many weeks, months and years to manifest. But they all start from one place, acid. It looks like this:

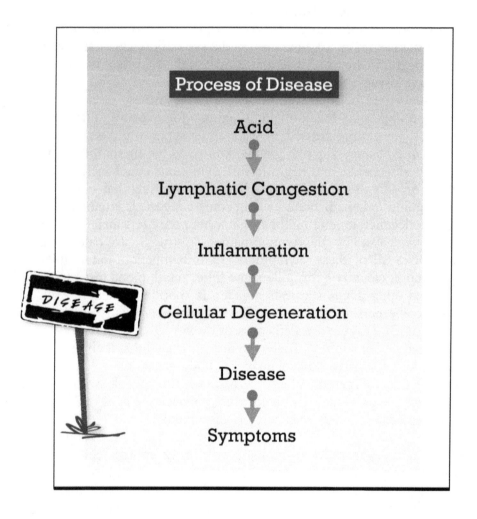

Acids break down tissue, literally. Conversely, if we *alkalize* the body, we can reverse the process of disease and witness symptoms fading away. Symptoms are often the *first* thing to subside, but this should NOT be mistaken for a cure. If that were so, then all of the suppressive pharmaceutical drugs of the world would be considered curative—which they are not. One should not be lulled into a false state of security and believe that the body is healed once symptoms are relieved. This will be discussed further in Chapter 8: "Steps to C.U.R.E."

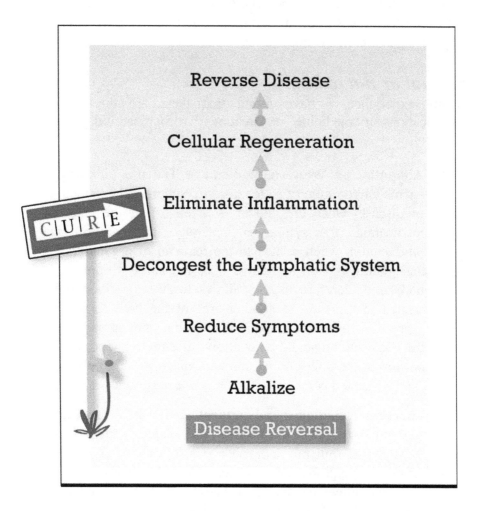

Reverse Disease

↑

Cellular Regeneration

↑

Eliminate Inflammation

↑

Decongest the Lymphatic System

↑

Reduce Symptoms

↑

Alkalize

Disease Reversal

C|U|R|E

Continuing to alkalize the body after symptoms disappear allows for lymphatic congestion to clear on a deeper level, inflammation to be quelled, cellular rejuvenation to occur, the return of cellular function and eventually the reversal of disease. It is in the alkalization of the cells and the decongestion of the lymphatic system (as well as supportive herbs and glandular tissues to be discussed in Chapter 8) which allows the human body to stand a chance of regenerating organs, tissues and glands, and reversing disease. Make no mistake, without alkalization there is no reversal of disease. At best you may just experience a cessation of symptoms, and as you have learned, suppressing symptoms is not healing.

To heal or not to heal

In my experience, I have found that there are three major classifications of "medicine" or "treatment" recognized today. They are as follows:

1. **Allopathy or Western medicine** – The use of chemical agents and/or surgery to temporarily suppress the symptoms of disease. Once the patient is taken off of the chemical medication, the symptoms generally reappear. Surgical intervention, when related to the removal of organs, tissues and glands as well as tumors does not cause a cure in the body and therefore usually allows for the condition being treated to "spread" to another area of the body (The term "spread" is misrepresented as disease does not spread across the body, but an acidic body allows disease to happen in any portion of the body). For example, cancer of the prostate can "spread" to the bone even if the prostate was removed.

2. **Functional medicine and natural medicine** – The use of "natural substances" (also known as isolated nutrients) such as vitamins, minerals, enzymes, probiotics, and the like to suppress symptoms of disease. Typically, many vials of blood are drawn and analyzed. These include standard CBC's (complete blood count), organ and gland profiles to vitamin and mineral levels and inflammatory markers. Isolated

nutrients are prescribed in an effort to "normalize" abnormal findings. Typically, once these nutritional products are discontinued, the symptoms tend to reappear; sometimes immediately, sometimes months or possibly years down the road. While the goal of these types of practices are to get to the "root" of the problem, they miss their mark in that they do not address the acid levels of the body or lymphatic congestion. Detoxification may be an objective, but they fall short and do not delve deep enough.

3. **Naturopathy; natural hygiene; traditional Chinese medicine** – The process of returning the body to a state of balance by creating a pristine internal environment. This is accomplished by removing processed, dead, acidic food and food-like substances from the diet as well as the removal of toxic substances from the lifestyle, including household cleaners and personal care products and replacing them with fresh, live, alkalizing plant-based foods and toxin-free products. Natural, whole herbs are introduced to support organs, tissues, and glands. These herbs are in their whole form and NOT isolated so that the body easily recognizes them, allowing them to be readily absorbed and utilized.

In my experience, supporting and promoting the functions of cells, tissues, organs, and glands with raw fruits and vegetables, herbs and glandular tissues as well as encouraging natural movement of the body (yoga, Tai Qi, Qi Gong etc.), incorporating daily meditation and encouraging one to reconnect with nature and their spiritual source which is the essence of Naturopathy and natural hygiene and is the most effective form of healing. Certain other modalities are often used as an adjunct to support the cleansing and healing process. These include: Acupuncture, tui na (Chinese body therapy and massage), cranial sacral therapy, lymphatic drainage massage, chiropractic, sound and vibrational healing, Reiki and numerous other natural healing therapies. Please refer to Chapter 9: "Supportive Treatment Modalities" for further information.

I have also found over the years, that it is EXTREMELY important to be humble in your beliefs about the form of treatment or medical approach you choose. Just because I have a strong feeling about one form over another, does not mean that I disregard the importance or abilities of other forms of treatment when used appropriately. In my own experience as a firefighter/EMT (emergency medical technician), as a practitioner of traditional Chinese medicine and as a patient, the ability to call on any of these branches of treatment at any given time is a gift that many people around the world do not have access to.

What I mean by that is this: In the 15 years I spent as a firefighter, I have never once thought to administer a fruit smoothie to someone who is in cardiac arrest or acupuncture to a gunshot victim. There are some very, very important times and places for Western medicine. Emergency medicine is one very important, irreplaceable aspect of western medicine. If you have been in a motor vehicle accident, had a heart attack, or a thyroid storm (just to mention a few), you must go to the ER! There are certain medical issues that must be handled by Western medicine first, for stabilization, before turning to a natural approach for long term reversal. Likewise, Western medicine, when used correctly, cannot be beat for diagnostics. Barring some of the dangers involved in certain diagnostics such as radiation or perforation, when not overused or improperly used Western medicine is quite savvy when it comes to blood tests, CAT scans, MRI, X-rays, and so on.

It's all in the genes
Time and time again, I am confronted with statements such as *"My doctor said it is genetic" "My father has diabetes so that is why I have it" and "High cholesterol runs in my family."*

The list of excuses for disease goes on and on, all of which serve to disempower the patient. Why do I say disempower? Well, if you were told by "experts" that there was something going on in your life that you had no control over, that no matter what you did, you could not change or improve, wouldn't you feel disempowered? Wouldn't you feel defeated? I know I would.

Now, I am not certain as to why a doctor would work to convince a patient that there is nothing they can do to lower cholesterol outside lack of knowledge or true understanding about where cholesterol comes from *(acid)* and why the body is so compelled to produce it in excess. Maybe the doctor does not want to put the time into explaining to the patient the cause of their elevated cholesterol. Maybe the doctor cannot bill the patient's insurance for such a discussion. Maybe the pharmaceutical companies who seem to run all of the continuing education seminars that doctors attend in order to keep their license do not want doctors competing for their massive profits. Maybe, maybe, maybe…At this point I cannot waste my time wondering why doctors continue this fairy tale about genes as the cause of disease. Instead I must move forward in helping people to understand why it is NOT! As science and statistics go, approximately <1% of all disease has a genetic only component. That means that the gene alone is the only causative factor of the disease in <1% of illnesses. Otherwise, all other disease processes have dual or multiple components. Let me say it another way.

A coconut has every genetic component it needs to become a coconut tree. After all, it is the seed of a coconut tree. If I dig a hole in my backyard (here in Florida), place the coconut in the hole, cover it with soil and water, within a few short weeks, the coconut will sprout and the life of a coconut tree will begin. It will not sprout into an apple tree or a peach tree or an oak tree. Its genes say that it is a coconut tree and therefore that is what it will be.

However, if I take my coconut on a trip to Canada, find a nice park, dig a hole and plant it, the coconut will not sprout, no matter how many weeks I wait. The coconut will never become a coconut tree. Even though it contains all of the genes needed to be a coconut tree, those genes will never be able to manifest because of one very important reason—the environment! Coconut trees do not grow in Canada. No matter how much water, sunshine, and love it receives, it will never sprout. Genes by themselves generally do not matter (though there are exceptions—for example, the chromosomal disorder that causes Down's syndrome is one example of a genetic issue that cannot be reversed by detoxification). Genes combined with environment matter. Alter the environment and you can turn the gene on or off! So my question to you…Is high cholesterol a genetic issue or an environmental one? Do you share the same genes or the same habits? I can ask the same regarding diabetes, heart disease, autoimmune diseases, or even cancer.

In his book *The China Study* (Campbell & Campbell, 1968), T. Colin Campbell, Ph. D. turned cancer on and off in rats just by increasing and decreasing the amount of casein (milk protein) that he fed them. As protein levels increased in the diet, cancer grew. Conversely, as dietary protein was decreased, cancerous tumors disappeared. It is on this premise that we venture into C.U.R.E. and learn how to Cultivate Unlimited Rejuvenating Energy.

Before moving forward, it is very important to address the fact that not all situations are able to be reversed. There are extenuating circumstances that stand in the way of healing. These circumstances include, but are not limited to:

- A high level of toxicity due to poisons, medications, chemotherapy, radiation, etc.

- A very weak body that has been sick for an extended period of time

- Severe genetic weakness

- A spirit's time to move on

"I believe as human beings we are out of balance, out of sync with the earth."

- Kevin Richardson

C|U|R|E *quotes*

chapter three
Chemistry 101: The Acid/Alkaline Tug of War

As a practitioner of traditional Chinese medicine (TCM) one of the first things that I learned was the concept of the duality of yin and yang. Yin and yang represent two opposing forces within the universe, our planet, nature, and within our bodies. Every aspect of life, chemistry, and for the purpose of this chapter, our bodies, can be divided into yin and yang endlessly. For example, the front of the body is yin while the back of the body is yang. The top of the front of the body is the yin half of the yin side while the bottom half of the front of the body is the yang half of the yin side. This can be confusing, but once you get it, you will forever look at living and inanimate objects based on their yin and yang aspects.

Yin represents the nutritive aspect of food, while yang is the energy that is gained from the nourishment. Yin is the coolness of the body that is balanced by yang, the heat or fire of the body. Yin is the fluid of the body, while yang is the force that moves the fluid. Yin is day and yang is night. Yin is female while yang is male. Yin regenerates while yang breaks down. Confusing? I thought so for the first year of traditional Chinese medicine (TCM) school! Eventually it all came together and the divisions of yin and yang proved to be the foundation for differential diagnoses and understanding illnesses in the human body from a Chinese medicine perspective.

According to TCM, the objective of these forces in the human body is to maintain balance (or as close to balance as possible) resulting in harmony and optimal health. This is known in biology as homeostasis.

The reason why I reference TCM and yin and yang is its relevance to the discussion of health and healing in the context of chemistry. You see, in chemistry, there are two opposing forces as well. They are known as acid and base—or for the purposes of nutrition, acid and alkaline. When these opposing forces are in their appropriate balance, for all intents and purposes, the human body remains healthy. But when these forces are out of balance, especially for a prolonged period of time, the human body deteriorates and becomes ill. Many times, regaining the balance of acid and alkaline forces in the body results in the healing of the illness. But there are certainly times when the imbalance has gone on so long and/or the genetic material of a person is so weak, that health cannot be regained. For me, this is the most distressing aspect of being a practitioner.

ACID/ALKALINE as it relates to diet

The process of determining how a food will react inside the human body (alkaline-forming or acid-forming) is done in a laboratory by incinerating a specific food and then analyzing the mineral content of the ash residue. If the mineral content is found to be highly alkaline, then it will have an alkaline effect on the human body. If it is found to be highly acidic, then it will have an acidic effect on the body. And, of course, there are varying degrees of acidity and alkalinity.

As we have undoubtedly observed in life, the human body is extremely resilient. Take into consideration the person who smokes cigarettes and drinks alcohol on a daily basis. They may go through their entire life with little to no obvious health issues until the very end when they are hospitalized with lung cancer and liver disease. The end may be an unhappy and harsh passage from life to death, even though the years prior were not particularly laden with doctor visits or hospital stays. Yet the person lived to be 70 years old. You may look at this and say, "70 years old, how can you complain about living that long?" But when we understand the fact that there are many communities of human beings throughout the world (Okinawa, Japan; Sardinia, Italy; Loma Linda, California; Nicoya, Costa Rica; Ikaria, Greece) whose residents are living for up to 115 years (not to mention the countless number of individuals all over the world) AND remain healthy, quite active, and devoid of prescription drugs or hospitalizations, then 70 years old no longer seems all that impressive.

The human body can sometimes tolerate a great deal of abuse, without any extreme or obvious hindrances, until the very end. That being said, it is in this resilience that the human body is constantly battling acid. The acid/alkaline tug of war happens on a moment to moment basis, non-stop, until the body just cannot battle anymore. Science calls this *homeostasis*—the tendency of the body to seek and maintain a condition of balance or equilibrium within its internal environment, even when faced with constant challenges and changes.

Let's take a closer look at an example of the acid/alkaline tug of war. For decades, milk and dairy products have been promoted as excellent food sources to build bone (until consumer advocacy groups began looking into the dairy industry claims and were able to debunk each one in court, forcing the milk industry to pull their falsely stated advertisements) due to its high calcium content. Yet the cells which make up bone, like all other structures and tissues of the human body, are comprised of more than just one material (in this case the material of focus is calcium). Calcium phosphate, magnesium, as well as two types of salts (carbonate and citrate sodium) are the inorganic compounds that make up bone. The nutrient factors effecting bone growth are:

1. Adequate levels of organic minerals and vitamins found in food sources

2. Availability of calcium and phosphorus

3. Intake of vitamins C, K, and B12

4. Production of vitamin D from sun exposure

Furthermore, when dairy is consumed, the ash residue that is left is acidic. This causes the triggering of a homeostatic response which releases a neutralizing substance that will allow the body to return to a neutral pH. The neutralizing substance is found in many tissues of the body including connective tissue, blood vessel walls AND bones. Can you guess the name of this neutralizing substance? If you guessed *calcium,* you are correct. The consumption of acid-forming foods will leave the body with no alternative but to release calcium into the bloodstream in an effort to neutralize acids and bring the body back to a balanced pH state. Therefore, the more acid-forming foods that you consume, the more the tissues of the body will have to release calcium.

Now, the mere fact that the body can do this, helps us to understand that we do need some acid in the diet. Our design *allows for* and *requires* us to consume a percentage of acid-forming food. Here again, we will use bone tissue to understand why.

Bone, like all tissues of the body, is in constant flux. Bone cells (osteocytes) are constantly dividing (osteogenesis) to create more bone, while other cells (osteoclasts) serve to break down bone tissue. This is how most tissues of the body work. Apoptosis (normal cell death) occurs so that new, stronger cells can replace old, weak ones. It is the acids in the diet that help this recycling process along.

The "tug of war" occurs when we ingest, inhale, or absorb (through the skin) more acid than the body can process and eliminate. In an effort to prevent excess destruction of cells, the body is continuously forced to pull neutralizers, such as calcium, from bones, blood vessel walls, and connective tissue (cartilage, tendons, ligaments and valves). The loss of calcium from these tissues results in health issues like osteopenia, osteoporosis, varicose and spider veins, aneurisms, connective tissue injuries and degenerative joint issues. Not to mention the acidic effects on all other tissues (glands, organs, and muscles) as discussed in the previous chapter.

The well-designed human body has an amazing ability to bring itself back to balance over and over and over again. But, as in all unstable relationships, eventually something's got to give! And when it does, it could be as benign as acne or as catastrophic as cancer.

It is important for us to understand that this tug of war will always persist. Yet, we have the ability to minimize it, sparing the body's resources for more important tasks and supplying it with all of the raw material it needs to carry them out. The best way to do this is to consume a diet that is mostly alkaline (at least 80%) and make wise decisions when choosing the acid-forming foods that our body needs.

As surprising as this may sound, even though I have been vegan for 24 years and have no intention otherwise, I truly believe that humans are not innately vegan. If we refer to Chapter 7, we can understand the basis from which I make this statement. Thus we can clearly see that the acidity of animal protein (in very small amounts) can actually have a beneficial effect in a long-term healthy diet. It's worth noting that these beneficial effects are of course present in a 100% plant-based diet.

But this is not a book about an optimal diet for a healthy body. It is not a book about the right food versus the wrong food. This is a book about how to wholly recover your health, whether you are seven months old or 70 years old. Today's health challenges are vast and far-reaching, affecting more and more people at younger and younger ages. Furthermore, we are not subject to just one illness at a time. In my acupuncture and detoxification practice, it is not unusual to meet someone with multiple autoimmune diseases, (the most I have personally seen were seven simultaneous autoimmune issues!) numerous degenerative/lifestyle issues (such as heart disease, diabetes and hypertension), or multiple types of cancer. It is also not unusual to see children with adult diseases and adults with diseases which render them near infantile. This book is for those people who have suffered at the hands of drugs and surgery and feel that enough is enough. This book is for those who understand the definition of insanity: If you keep doing what you've always done and expect a different result, you are nuts! This book is for you if you are ready to go way, way outside the box and bring yourself back to nature. That is the acid/alkaline tug of war. That is the war we rage on disease. That is the internal struggle of comprehending that nature knows best, versus falling into the same old social patterns that led you to ignore your health to begin with. This book is a gift for you to truly understand the life giving force of alkalization versus the life robbing power of acids.

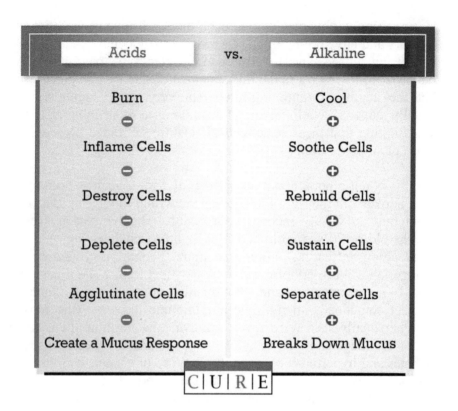

Acids	vs.	Alkaline
Burn		Cool
⊖		⊕
Inflame Cells		Soothe Cells
⊖		⊕
Destroy Cells		Rebuild Cells
⊖		⊕
Deplete Cells		Sustain Cells
⊖		⊕
Agglutinate Cells		Separate Cells
⊖		⊕
Create a Mucus Response		Breaks Down Mucus

C | U | R | E

Picture watching your favorite DIY (do-it-yourself) show. You will inevitably see the host of the show choosing an old home, antique car, or worn-out piece of furniture to "make new" again. The dilapidated item may be old, dingy, weathered, and falling apart, its foundation cracked or hood rusted, but the host promises a rejuvenation of grand proportions.

Step one would be to sand down, chisel away, or acid wash the broken down piece of furniture, rusted car or weathered floor. After all, you have to get rid of the old before introducing the new! That is what acid does in the body; it breaks down, destroys, and does away with cells and tissue. We accept that as part of life. After all, cells live and die (apoptosis) on a daily basis. Just as in your home, lights go out, carpets wear down and window screens tear, and so too does this occur in the body. Yet ask yourself, would you ever consider not replacing the light in your stairwell or the carpet where your baby crawls?

So what happens to a house that you neglect? How long can it last on its own if it is given no attention, no care, or upkeep? Over time, the elements will take their toll on the house and it will break down. This too occurs in your body on a cellular level. Consuming processed foods, dead animal flesh, and heaps of sugar can inevitably destroy cells to a point of no return. In an old house, it takes someone who can see the potential in the "bones" of the structure and who is willing to put in the time and effort, to bring the structure back to life. In regard to your health, you must see the innate potential your body has for healing and then be willing to do the work! Simply stated, in the human body, this means alkalizing, rejuvenating, and regenerating tissue. This is possible but you *must* take the time NOW. You must care NOW. You must be willing to change NOW. Most importantly, you must care more about yourself than I care about you.

As you eliminate the acid (weather damage) and begin to alkalize your cells (new roof) you regain the health and vitality that you believed you lost just because you became older. You begin to truly understand that what you do today ALWAYS affects your tomorrow. Thus if you make positive (alkaline) choices today, tomorrow inevitably must be better.

Everything you eat or drink will build cells up or break cells down. So in the battle of acid versus alkalinity the question remains…Which foods are alkalinizing to the body and which are acidic? What percentage of each should you consume? The answers lie below.

When detoxifying, the answer is go big or go home! 100% of your diet should be alkaline. That means fruit and vegetables (with a very strong emphasis on fruit) in their raw state. While there are times cooked food is allowed, the most rapid detoxification results occur on a raw diet. The details will be presented later in Chapter 8: "Steps to C.U.R.E." along with answers to your questions, e.g. raw food, protein needs, and the fear of fruit and too much sugar.

In the meantime, I leave you with this thought...Making food choices based on MACRO-nutrients (protein, fats, and carbohydrates) alone is insanity! Looking at nutrition this way is missing a tremendous piece of the picture. There is so much more to nutrition. There is far more to feeding, nourishing, and healing your body. Putting your attention on macronutrients is a distraction from truth. Truth is found in the totality of living food. Not only in the protein, fat and carbohydrate aspects of food, but in the vitamins, minerals, enzymes, water, and above all—life giving energy, vibration and LIFE-FORCE only found in raw fruit and vegetables!

There is no substitution for raw fruits and vegetables. In the tug of war between acid and alkaline forces in the human body, these are the foods that tip the scales in the direction of the greatest healing potential. Chapter 13 will provide an extensive list of food and where it lies on the acid alkaline scale. Please note that NOT ALL ALKALINE FOODS are allowed during detoxification.

"To eat is a necessity,
  but to eat intelligently is an art."

- Francois de La Rochefoucauld

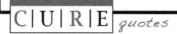

chapter four
Where do I get my protein?

This chapter was written by my husband, Anthony Serpico. Following several months of detoxification to reverse high blood pressure (which started following ankle surgery due to a motocross accident), Anthony decided to get back into body building. At the time he was almost 50 years old and had been vegan for 20 years. Although, I must admit, we were in many ways acid vegans. While we did consume fruits and vegetables, we were also big fans of nuts and nut butters, beans, rice, quinoa, cereal, pasta, and anything made with them! So, once Anthony had reversed his high blood pressure, he was challenged with the task of building muscle on a fruit and vegetable diet. After all, he wanted to maintain an alkaline state, but also desired a strong, lean, muscular body. And according to all of the body building magazines, YouTube videos and blogs he researched, you HAD TO consume large quantities of protein to accomplish this. The best form, according to the pundits of course, being animal protein. Luckily, Anthony knew enough not to sacrifice his health for his muscles. He began to research the amount of protein he would need to build a strong body and how much of that protein could be found in the alkaline diet that reversed his high blood pressure.

As we took our morning walks with our Weimaraner (yes, we are the only vegans who own a hunting dog!), Nero, Anthony would excitingly report his research to me. I found this information so intriguing and important that I asked him to write it down so that I could share it with my patients. While some of the foods mentioned in this chapter are not incorporated during detoxification, they are certainly acceptable in moderate amounts after detox. The end result is as follows:

Where do you get your protein?

As a vegan this is the question I most often hear. The reasoning is as follows: as a vegan you don't eat any meat, poultry, fish or dairy, and therefore could not possibly be getting sufficient quantities of high quality protein. As we shall see, nothing could be further from the truth. Not only is it possible to obtain all the protein necessary as a vegan, I would go further and argue that *plant based protein is actually superior to animal protein.* So, let's get started investigating this non-issue.

How much protein do we need?

The answer to this question provides us with a starting point for understanding protein needs. Unfortunately, there is no definitive optimal daily protein requirement. The short answer is no one really knows precisely how much protein an individual needs for optimal health. There are guidelines that identify minimal requirements, but "minimal" does not imply optimal. Those with sedentary lifestyles are believed to have lower protein requirements than active individuals. It's also generally accepted that high intensity training increases protein requirements. The operative words being "generally" and "believed." I hate to muddy the waters so much, but the fact is there's still a quite a bit that is unknown about protein metabolism. That being said, there is a lot that is known and we can use this knowledge to guide us along. So, back to the question, "How much protein do we need?" Generally accepted guidelines suggest that healthy adults should consume between 0.5 and 1.5 grams of protein per kilogram of lean bodyweight. So, for an adult weighting 150 lbs. that would be between ~34 and ~105 grams. That's quite the range! You might ask, "What's the right number", but you already know the answer to that question. For our discussion let's just settle on 0.8 grams of protein per kilogram of bodyweight. This represents a reasonable daily intake that meets the recommended minimum daily allowance, yet is not so high as to present any risk to healthy adults.

As wide as the above variations are, I have seen advice doled out suggesting individuals should consume 1 or even 1.5 grams of protein per pound of lean body mass. For me, that would be between 130 and 195 grams. I have also witnessed NDs and other holistic healers use ultra-low protein detox-diets with great success in curing difficult chronic illnesses.

As an interesting side note, the amount of protein in mothers' milk is ~2 percent of calories.

What are essential amino acids?

First, a little background. Every cell in the body is comprised of proteins. Amino acids are the substances that make up protein. Our bodies use 22 amino acids to synthesize the ~50,000 different proteins we need to be healthy. Of the 22 amino acids, there are nine that are labeled essential. An essential amino acid is one that cannot be synthesized by the body from other available resources, and therefore must be supplied by one's diet.

You may have heard of branched chain amino acids, also known as BCAAs. There are three BCAAs, all of which are among the nine essential amino acids. They are:

- Leucine

- Isoleucine

- Valine

For this discussion, let's ignore what technically distinguishes a BCAA from a regular amino acid. So, why do I bring them up? BCAAs account for ~33% of the essential amino acids found in muscle proteins. There is a concern, mostly among men trying to build muscle, that a failure to consume these essential elements will hinder their development.

So, where do you get your protein?

I'm glad you asked. In this section I am going to shine a light on the vegan protein sources that I use both during and after detox, so expect the variety to be broader than when you begin to detox.

The plant kingdom provides many excellent sources. Just about any plant, nut, or seed that you eat will provide ample protein, but let's go over a few of the more interesting options.

- Hemp seeds

- Chia seeds

- Dark green leafy vegetables, e.g. chard, spinach, kale, collards

- Sprouted sunflower seeds

- Quinoa

- Pea sprouts

Hemp seeds

It is quite possible that there is no better source of protein than hemp seed. By weight, they are one of the most protein dense foods in the world. One ounce (28 g) contains an impressive 9 g of protein. That's 30% protein by weight. This puts virtually all animal based sources of protein to shame, but this is only the beginning. By taking a closer look, we find that the real power in hemp protein is not in its quantity, as impressive as it is, but in its protein quality. Hemp seed protein is ~67% globulin edistin, and ~33% globulin albumin, which makes hemp a protein that is readily available in a form quite similar to that which is found in blood plasma. Of course, hemp seeds contain all nine essential amino acids. In addition, hemp seeds also contain the essential fatty acids omega-3 and omega-6 in the proper ratios. Hemp is not a low calorie food; at ~160 calories per ounce it is fairly dense, but don't let that scare you off, hemp seeds are a phenomenal source of protein.

As an added benefit, most hemp is organic. Being a weed, it is a tough, resilient plant that requires little attention when grown in suitable conditions. Pesticides and herbicides are rarely needed to successfully grow hemp.

Sprouted Sunflower Seeds

Sprouted sunflowers are truly impressive; their nutritional numbers are off the charts. I encourage you to look into them further. For our discussion we are focused on protein, and here too, sprouted sunflowers don't disappoint. As one of the richest sources of protein, one ounce (28 g) of sprouted sunflower seeds contains an impressive 6.5 grams of protein, ~25% protein by weight. Sprouted sunflower seeds are quite low in calories, yet rich in many nutrients and minerals.

A mere 3.5 ounces of sprouted sunflower seeds contains a whopping ~23 grams of protein! The same amount of:

- Chicken breast meat contains just slightly more protein at ~26 grams

- Hamburger patty: ~24 grams protein

- Most cuts of beef: ~24 grams of protein

- Tuna: ~26 grams of protein

- Most fish fillets or steaks contain ~22 grams of protein

Dark green leafy vegetables, e.g. chard, spinach, kale, collards

Often overlooked for their protein value, dark leafy green vegetables contain high concentrations of protein per calorie. For example, 30 grams of spinach contain only ~7 calories but have ~1 gram of protein. As a general rule, five ounces of dark leafy greens contain ~4 grams of protein at around 40 calories. While this may not seem like much, it compares very favorably to animal protein sources. For example, one cup of 2% milk contains ~122 calories and ~8 grams of protein. For the same 122, calories you would get over 15 grams of protein from spinach. That's nearly double the calorie to protein ratio. And contrary to popular belief, virtually all dark leafy greens provide a complete source of protein that contains all nine essential amino acids.

Our focus on protein ignores all of the other health benefits found in dark greens, but that's a topic for another article.

Quinoa (pronounced KEEN-WAH)

You might ask "what is Quinoa?" Quinoa is the seed of a green leafy plant that is indigenous to South America. It is often referred to as a grain but I believe it is technically the fruit of an herb. The great thing about quinoa is that it can serve as a direct replacement to rice. Wherever and however you use rice, you can use quinoa in its place. As a protein source, quinoa is quite valuable. It is a complete protein that contains all nine essential amino acids, it is gluten free, easy to digest, and high in fiber. One ounce of quinoa contains ~4 grams of protein and ~110 calories. One cup of cooked quinoa contains ~9 grams of protein.

Chia Seeds

Chia seed are comprised of ~20-30% protein, ~35% oil, and ~25% fiber. Chia is gluten-free, very low in sodium, and has a very good omega-3 to omega-6 ratio. Of course, they are a complete source of protein, providing all nine essential amino acids in an easily digestible form. Chia is also a great source of soluble fiber. At ~140 calories, one ounce (~28 g) of Chia seeds contain ~5 g of protein. I could extoll the virtues of chia seeds for pages, but we are focusing on protein.

Let's compare one ounce of chia seeds to one egg, often considered an excellent source of protein. One large egg (~46 g) contains ~90 calories with ~6 g of protein. Both eggs and chia seeds contain all essential amino acids. It turns out the calorie to protein ratio of an egg is a bit better than chia seeds, but at what cost? An egg gets ~70% of its calories from fat and contains a whopping 220 mg of cholesterol (The RDA for cholesterol is 300 mg). So let's put this in perspective, if you eat just two eggs you will have only gotten ~12 g of protein at a cost of ~440 mg of cholesterol. According to the RDA, you're already way over your daily cholesterol limit and should stop consuming any more foods containing cholesterol. Or to put it another way, you need to stop eating additional meat, poultry, fish, and dairy.

Pea Sprouts

Pea sprouts are another great source of protein. A 3.5 ounce serving contains ~9 grams of protein at 128 calories. That's about the same protein to calorie ratio as an egg, except pea sprouts contain 0 mg of cholesterol and only 1% fat (non-saturated). And, like virtually all sprouts, pea sprouts are nutrient dense.

Do plant based foods contain "complete" proteins?

First, we should answer the question of which properties a food must have in order to qualify as a "complete" protein source. Unfortunately, the answer to this depends on who you talk to, although it probably shouldn't. In any case, below are the two most common definitions, with the latter being more restrictive.

- A food must contain at least all nine essential amino acids in order to be a complete protein source.

- A food must contain at least all nine essential amino acids in the proper quantities in order to qualify as a complete protein source. The theory being that if a food contains one or more amino acids in quantities below some threshold, then the body will be unable to synthesize protein from that food source.

It doesn't really matter which you choose to believe because neither present a dietary challenge for vegetarians. As for the first definition, it appears to me that virtually all plant based foods contain all nine essential amino acids. I was unable to find any fruit or vegetable that did not qualify as a complete protein source based on this definition.

The second definition is a bit more nuanced. According to this, even if a food contains all nine essential amino acids, it may still not qualify as a complete source of protein because it may lack one or more of the amino acids in sufficient quantities. However, this definition is unrealistic about how it considers food consumption and protein metabolism. Who eats a single serving of a food in isolation over a day? To illustrate my point, let's consider peaches, not exactly known as a power packed source of protein. One large peach, ~175 grams, contains ~2 grams of protein. Of course, it contains all nine essential amino acids, but, according to conventional nutritional thinking, at least seven of these amino acids are lacking in sufficient quantities in order to consider a peach a complete protein. But what if I eat two peaches; will I then have consumed enough of the seven lacking amino acids? The answer is yes. Obviously, this notion of needing to consume foods that are complete proteins in and of themselves or the combining of complimentary foods is unnecessary. All you need to do in order to consume sufficient quantities of protein is to eat the proper number of calories needed to maintain your proper body weight.

Let's take this peach example one step further. Again, a large peach contains ~2 grams of protein at ~68 calories. I weigh 150 pounds and require ~1700 calories a day to maintain my bodyweight. If all I ate were peaches (1700 calories worth of peaches) I would be consuming ~50 grams of protein a day. That's still right at the ~55 grams suggested for someone my weight.

Let me be clear, I am very much in favor of eating a wide variety of plant based foods, for a number of reasons. But from the perspective of protein, it's not really necessary.

Making dietary choices
This section focuses on the protein component of plant based food sources. However, this is really an overly simplistic way of evaluating the quality of any particular food. To isolate a specific compound in a food, in this case protein, and make judgments as to the quality of one's selection ignores everything else about the particular food. This is not a rational way to make dietary choices. For example, the dairy industry loves to remind people that milk contains copious amounts of calcium, and by extension, must therefore be good for bones. But it has been clearly established that milk is, in fact, quite bad for bones. Why? Well, like virtually all animal protein sources, milk acidifies the body's pH which in turn triggers your body to perform a correction to rebalance. It turns out calcium is an excellent acid neutralizer and the biggest store of calcium in the body are your bones. So the very same calcium that our bones need to stay healthy is depleted in order to neutralize the acidifying effect of milk. My point is that food must be evaluated in its totality. In the first paragraph of this chapter I stated that I believed plant based protein to be superior to animal protein. I believe this to be the case not because I think plant protein is in and of itself somehow superior to animal protein but rather because of all their other qualities.

My own experience

I have been a vegan for over 24 years and have never experienced symptoms of protein deficiency, and I make no special effort to regulate my protein intake. I simply eat a variety of fruits and vegetables along with occasional grains, nuts, and seeds.

From the ages of 26 through 37 I was involved in the sport of bodybuilding, a sport many would say increases one's protein needs. When I was 29 I switched from a typical animal based diet to a vegan diet. Not only did the switch not impede my performance, I believe that in the long run it actually contributed to my development. My body seemed to better manage the stresses of heavy weightlifting. Recovery times appeared to shorten and I suffered fewer nagging low-level injuries. For the past eleven years I have been busy participating in the sport of motocross/supercross racing, and at no time did I feel at a disadvantage due to my diet. Actually, it's quite the opposite, I believe being a vegan has allowed me to perform at a high level in this very demanding sport. In motocross it is inevitable that injuries will come, but my body's ability to recuperate seemed no different from when I was much younger. Again, this is something I attribute to my diet.

My typical diet

While the graphic on the following page is not my diet during the detoxification process, I thought it might be interesting to take a look at my typical day to see what food sources I am getting my protein from. As I stated earlier, I don't make any special effort to regulate or monitor my own protein intake. This is actually the first time that I will be adding up the actual grams of protein in my diet. Of course, my daily diet varies and does not exactly follow what I did today, which is what I wrote down, but it does follow a very similar pattern, especially during the work week.

1 — Wake up and have 1 cup of coconut water and peach or some other fruit ---------- 3 grams

2 — Morning shake consisting of 1 oz of almonds, 1 oz, of hemp seeds, 1 banana, water and ice. I sweeten with stevia. Sometimes I include cacao beans ---------- 17 grams

3 — About two hours later I have 1 banana ---------- 1 grams

4 — About 1 hour later I have ~ 2 cups of grapes and ~1 cup of strawberries, or some similar mix of fruit ---------- 3 grams

5 — About 1 hour later I have ~ 2 oz of sprouted sunflower seeds and ~1 oz of dandelion or similar leafy green and 1 cup of coconut water ---------- 16 grams

6 — Short time later I have 1 avocado with 1/2 oz of hemp seeds and 12 oz of fresh vegetable juice. ---------- 10 grams

7 — About an hour later I have 5 oz of mixed greens (red chard, green chard, arugula, spinach, tat soi, etc.) ---------- 4 grams

8 — 1/2 cup of quinoa with 1-1/2 cups of steamed mixed vegetables ---------- 11 grams

TOTAL Protein -------- 65 grams

0.94 protein grams per Kg of bodyweight

C|U|R|E

Now that you know my typical diet when I am not detoxing, let's take a look at a menu during detoxification. Keep in mind that my workout routine changed dramatically during those 12 weeks as per

Dr. Morse's instructions. While he would have preferred that I refrain from working out all together, we compromised on a much reduced schedule.

Of course, my daily diet does not exactly follow what I did today, which is what I wrote down below, but it does follow a very similar pattern, especially during the work week.

Prior to detox I worked out 3–4 days per week at high intensity. That included weight lifting, running on the beach and dragging sand bags. Once I began detox I decreased my routine to only two days per week with dramatically lower intensity. The sand bags were out and running often morphed into a brisk walk. There were certainly days that I felt I could do more, but I the chance that I might pay for it the next day in the form of low energy or even fatigue kept me on the straight and narrow.

In regard to the diet, not only did I feel it was sustainable and satisfying, it was no more difficult than my non-detox diet. The best part was that I lost very little size or strength and when I did return to my normal workout routine I felt an incredible sense of vitality! Within a few shorts weeks I felt stronger than before detox. It is also important to note that I did not reduce my schedule at the office. I have been a software engineer for 30 years and during the detoxification process I had no issue with focus, concentration, or productivity.

The photo on the reverse page was taken at the *Superhero Scramble,* (a four-mile race with 14 obstacles and lots of mud) just 2 months after completing my 12-week detoxification program. I was 50 years old, vegan for nearly 20 years and felt better than ever placing in the top 10% of all age groups. I have run over a dozen obstacle course races since then, some of which took me through ice water, electric shock, freezing temperatures and sizzling deserts up to 13 miles. I feel that my diet and what I learned from detoxification has allowed me to not only participate in these races consistently place in the top 5-10%. Best of all, I find that my body recovers effortlessly afterward.

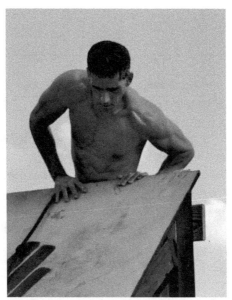

Photo taken 2 months after 12-week detox
24 years vegan
Age 50

"And when you crush an apple with your teeth,
say to it in your heart:
  Your seeds shall live in my body,
  And the buds of your tomorrow shall blossom
    in my heart,
  And your fragrance shall be my breath,
  And together we shall rejoice through all
    the seasons."

- Kahlil Gibran

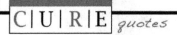 C | U | R | E *quotes*

chapter five
Fruit, glorious fruit!

I know what you are thinking, so let's get it out of the way right here and now. You have likely flipped through this book before purchasing it, and while the cover, title, and chapters intrigued you, there is one part of this book that concerns you. After everything that you have heard and read regarding diets, natural therapies, healing the body, weight loss, cancer, diabetes, etc. you are quite certain that you *should not* be eating "so much" fruit! After all, fruit is high in sugar, it will make you gain weight, and it feeds cancer! Why, fruit may be one of the scariest foods on the planet! *Right?* Wrong! Calm down, take a moment and *breathe*. All will be ok, I promise.

No matter how many points I make about the human as a species and how our anatomy dictates our diet, there is going to be that small percentage of people who call this *"the same old tired argument."* I am confident about this because I have had that discussion with "those people" and I am here to tell you, it's okay. Keep believing what you will. I am not here to change the world (although I would love to!). Instead, my purpose is to help one person at a time to regain their health and vitality. As my friend and well-known raw food nutritionist Fred Bisci, PhD once said, *"I don't want you to believe me or anyone else, I only ask that you try it and see how you feel."*

It is so true that I have to say it again. Fruit, glorious fruit! It is the stuff that dreams are made of. To be able to eat something so delicious, juicy, and sweet is a gift from God (or nature if you prefer). It is its sugar that draws us to it and for good reason. Fruit provides us with endless amounts of nutrition, but let us start with this tasty treat's most controversial component: Sugar.

Fruit contains two types of sugar, fructose (approximately 55%) and glucose (approximately 45%), whereas table sugar contains sucrose. Sucrose must be broken down by the enzyme beta-fructosidase which separates sucrose into its individual sugar units, glucose (50%) and fructose (50%). While fruit and table sugar both contain comparable ratios of fructose and glucose, that is where their similarity ends, in terms of how the human body uses them. Let's compare strawberries to strawberry ice cream.

For right now we are going to ignore the obvious and not discuss other nutrients found in fruit. The focus here is on sugar. First, fruit tends to have less sugar by volume than foods containing sucrose. For example, a half cup of strawberries contains 3.5 grams of sugar whereas a half cup of strawberry ice cream contains 15 grams.

While gram for gram the percentage of fructose to glucose is virtually the same, there are some things you need to know. Fructose breaks down in the liver and does not provoke an insulin response. Glucose starts to break down in the stomach and requires the release of insulin into the bloodstream to be metabolized completely. The fiber that naturally occurs in all fruit dramatically slows down the release of glucose into the blood stream, causing an extremely minor insulin response. (This means that the body has more time to use up glucose as fuel before storing it as fat. Even dried fruit, known for its high sugar content, has enough fiber and nutrients to avoid an undue spike in blood sugar.) Sucrose, found in ice cream, cake, soda and candy contains little to no fiber resulting in a tremendous blood sugar spike followed by an insulin dump and subsequent blood sugar crash. This process causes great harm to a diabetic, as opposed to fruit, which when given during the detoxification process (and beyond) along with the appropriate herbs, will result in a stabilization of blood sugar. (Keep in mind that there is much more for you to learn about detoxification, rejuvenation, and the use of herbs which will be discussed beyond this chapter, to help reverse diabetes and other processes of disease). In the case of type I diabetes, when one is detoxing and consuming fruit on a daily basis there is a possibility that some fruit may cause a temporary spike in blood sugar. If this occurs, you may remove that particular fruit for the time being. Eventually you should be able to include it in your diet. (Type I diabetics may never be able to come off of insulin completely, but they will be able to significantly reduce the amount of insulin needed.) And finally, the fear of fruit for diabetics during detoxification and beyond can be put to rest.

Sugar has a power to draw us in like no other component of our diet, and for good reason. Sugar or carbon (carbohydrates) provides the energy that drives us. More specifically, the energy that drives our cells. While the human body can use protein or fat as energy, its first choice are carbohydrates. Carbohydrates are the simplest source of energy and every cell of your body primarily relies on sugar to operate. Nature makes choosing the right foods to provide your body with the optimal balance of sugar and fiber easy by making fruit abundant, varied and delicious. When you are considering going for a run, taking a 90-minute yoga class or squatting your rear end into oblivion, fruit will provide the greatest source of energy with a minimal amount of digestive effort, packaged perfectly for transport!

One of the greatest concerns I hear from people is that of sugar and it ability to "feed cancer." Well, it is true. Sugar, including fruit sugar does in fact, feed cancer cells. But as I said before, sugar feeds *all* cells. There are approximately 100 trillion cells that make up the human body. Of those 100 trillion cells, a cancerous tumor makes up a very tiny fraction. So to avoid sugar in an effort to starve a cancer tumor will result in starving the entire body. It is not only crazy to avoid sugar in the diet, but impossible. That is unless you decided to eat only animal flesh and eggs. You see, everything else - grains (maltose), dairy (galactose), nuts (sucrose), beans (glucose), and vegetables (glucose) contains sugar! Furthermore, there is absolutely no research to support that eating a diet of only dead animal flesh will serve to reverse cancer (or any other disease for that matter). In fact, virtually ALL Western medicine studies regarding diet and cancer specifically recommend that you increase fruits and vegetables in your diet and decrease animal protein. There is hardly a cancer found today that cannot be linked to diet.

Another glorious fact about fruit is its ability to hydrate our cells better than any other food including water. Today, most tap water is laden with toxins from chlorine to residue of pharmaceutical drugs as well as fluoride and arsenic. Bottled water is typically just" filtered" tap water and if truly bottled from a spring, it is packaged in a plastic bottle which will leach God knows what into our water.

Commercial water, when tested, tends to fall on the acidic side of chemistry and if you are lucky enough to find water that is in alkaline and in glass bottles, you may not be able to afford it on a daily basis.

Conversely, fruit contains the purest and most abundant amount of alkaline water there is. Okay, maybe the water of a glacier is just as pure, but it doesn't have everything fruit does. When eating a diet high in fruit, it is virtually unheard of to feel thirsty.

Wait! What about weight?

Once again, understanding that your cells require sugar for energy is step one to welcoming fruit back into your diet. But wait, there's more! By weight, the energy that fruit provides for your cells is some of the lowest calorie, highest nutrition foods you could eat. Fruit's ability to alkalize the body as well as detoxify and purge waste plays an important part in weight loss. Excess weight is not just about calories in and calories out. Nor is it about one macro nutrient. Fat cells hold on to toxins in an effort to protect the more important cells (vital organs and endocrine glands) from harm. Fruit is the most effective detoxifier that nature provides. The ability of fruit to alkalize the body and purge toxic waste will rapidly escort fat from the body as well.

And then there is...everything else. We have been trained (via media, medicine, and nutrition experts) to look at our food from one dimension. Yes, each fruit and vegetable in its raw, whole state provides the body with a multitude of micronutrients, enzymes, and phytochemicals, as well as protein, fat, and carbohydrates. Yet raw fruit provides us with even more than that!

When we look at food solely in terms of its nutritional content, we miss an enormous piece of the detoxification, healing, and regeneration puzzle. Every living thing on this planet gives off electromagnetic energy in the form of vibration. This energy is rated in units called Angstroms. Food in its raw state gives off a higher amount of energy than cooked food. Most importantly, fresh (and even more so freshly picked) raw fruit has the highest amount of angstroms compared to any other food! The human species requires a minimum of 6000 to 7000 angstroms of systemic energy at all times just to maintain life and a basic level of health. Between 4500 and 5200 angstroms, the body becomes susceptible to disease. At that level, degeneration of tissue will continue opening the door to autoimmune issues, heart disease, or cancer. If you are in a diseased or debilitated state, your body will require much more than 7000 angstroms to recover. That is where fruit shines! Like the sun that our earth revolves around, fruit is the center of our nutritional solar system, sustaining all that is life. No longer do we look at food for its mere protein, fat, or carbohydrate content. Choosing a food based on its vitamin or mineral profile is passé. But choosing food for its ability to raise our internal energy and build cellular power and longevity is what this book is all about.

Understanding the endless benefits of whole, raw fruit brings us to an awareness that vitamins and minerals in the form of a supplement is dead. Cooked vegetable matter or animal flesh is dead. Canned, packaged, and preserved food is dead. So how can you regenerate living cells with dead food, lacking in vital energy and vibration? You can't.

When cleaning the lymphatic system, it is the astringing power of fruit (especially grapes, lemons, limes) that literally pulls toxic lymph from the spaces between the cells, freeing it so that it may ultimately be removed from the body. Fruit specifically aids in the regeneration of adrenal glands as well as the neurological system. The power of fruit runs deep and we are likely only scratching the surface of nature's perfect food. I do not have enough pages in this book or knowledge to list all of the amazing edible fruit in the world. In your detox journey and beyond, I encourage you to explore the bounty that God/nature has given us. Please abandon your comfort zone of apples and bananas and discover...

- Monstera delisiosa

- Jack fruit

- Durian

- Egg fruit

- Sour sop

- Dragon fruit

- Passion fruit

- Coconut

- Mangosteen

- Lychee

- Custard apple

- Guava

"This too shall pass."

- unknown Persian Sufi poet

C | U | R | E *quotes*

Chapter 6
The Process of Elimination

There is no question that this is a crappy subject which is typically discussed by those over the age of 65. But when it comes to optimal health, the process of elimination is an extremely crucial subject. And, as they say, someone has to talk about it.

Elimination of waste is actually a very broad topic, encompassing not only the elimination of metabolic wastes from the cells into the lymphatic system, but also the elimination of digestive waste via the colon. As a health care practitioner, when it comes to the topic of eliminating digestive waste, I have heard it all. For example, the bathroom habits of someone with irritable bowel syndrome (IBS) can range from 5 to10 bowel movements a day, to the opposite extreme where they can skip having a bowel movement for one or more days. Conversely, those with chronic constipation may not have a normal bowel movement for several days or even weeks! I once had a patient who told me she only had a bowel movement once every two weeks, and yet her doctor said that was "her normal." I am literally on the verge of exploding when I hear such ignorance from a medical professional!

Shortly after a newborn baby comes into the world, it has a bowel movement. The waste that the baby passes is called meconium. Meconium is a combination of mucus, amniotic fluid, bile, water, and cellular waste from the lining of the intestines. Once meconium is passed, the pathway of elimination is open. As the infant begins to breast feed, this pathway remains open and the child is expected to have 4 to 8 bowel movements per day. If the baby continues to be fed mother's breast milk, they will continue to eliminate waste regularly and with ease. The waste should be generally easy to clean up after with little foul odor. But oftentimes, as the child gets older, the habits of elimination change and parents are commonly informed by the doctor that this change is "normal."

My question: Why is this normal? Is it because doctors see children devolve in their eliminative habits so often that they mistake *common* for *normal*? Is there a natural reason why we eat more food as we get older and eliminate less? The truth is that there is nothing normal or natural about humans eliminating less volumes of waste as they get older. It is our diet and virtually just our diet that causes humans to stop eliminating waste 2–4 times a day.

If a child is lucky, their mother will breast feed them until 12 months of age and they will never be exposed to highly processed baby formula, nor the milk of another species (e.g. cow, goat etc.). Between 4–6 months of age, solid food is introduced. Solid food should be defined as fresh and minimally processed, for example, by mashing with a fork or by a food processor. Fruit is most desirable, and should remain raw, while being fed in accordance with the basic food combination chart (see appendix). The introduction of vegetables can wait until fruit has been given for 1–2 weeks so that the digestive system can adjust. Unfortunately, vegetables have to be lightly steamed or juiced raw before consumption. Again, food combination rules should always be followed. As the child gets older and a variety of foods are introduced, it is imperative for proper eliminative health (as well as general health) that processed foods ARE NOT INTRODUCED into the diet. This may seem harsh, difficult, or challenging because it requires some planning and preparation, not to mention some battles with friends and family, but it is the greatest gift that you can give your child. Remember, just because a child can eventually put their thumb and index fingers together, grasp an object, and reach their mouth, doesn't mean we should put a Cheerio in from of them. Getting them hooked on processed grain products is not healthy nor supportive of proper digestion.

Processed food is one of the greatest disasters to befall the digestive tract in modern times. These foods are high in salt, sugar, and grains which not only acidify the body, but greatly congest both the small and large intestines. This congestion causes a decrease in the body's ability to eliminate waste, as well as mild to severe malabsorption.

Malabsorption can be explained as such: The walls of the small intestines can be likened to the screen on your bedroom window. Its purpose is to allow air to pass through while keeping pests out. Fresh air flows through the tiny holes of the screen much like molecules of nutrition pass through the intestinal wall and into the blood stream. But if I were to spread a thick layer of mud across the screen, it would stick between the tiny spaces, preventing air from flowing through freely. The breeze could be diminished by 25, 50, or even 90%! In much the same way the absorption of nutrition is greatly reduced after years of a processed food (and dairy) laden diet.

As thick and sticky processed food makes its way through the microvilli in the small intestine, it adheres to the walls, blocking the microscopic spaces between the villi. This can eventually lead to damage of the villi and malabsorption of nutrition. The reduced transit time of waste through the large intestine causes constipation (less than two bowel movements per day) which can eventually lead to intestinal issues such as colitis, IBS, Crohn's, polyps or cancer. Over time, the lack of proper elimination will cause a systematic toxic buildup which can result in headaches, allergies, sinus inflammation, skin issues, auto immune diseases, chronic degenerative diseases (e.g. heart disease, diabetes, hypertension), and cancers. Malabsorption due to the improper elimination of waste, congestion of the intestines, and destruction of the mucosa and villi will lead to a host of nutrient deficiency syndromes too numerous to list. The implications of malabsorption are far and wide. Beyond the previously stated ailments and diseases, one must also consider a correlation between a congested digestive tract and a lack of nutrient absorption, which may cause a slew of cognitive issues such as ADD, ADHD, OCD, Alzheimer's, and dementia as well as emotional issues such as depression, anxiety, and aggression.

As you can see, the body's ability to eliminate waste is a critical process. This process is required to function correctly for virtually every aspect of our health. Dismissing one's inability to eliminate waste daily as being "normal" is irresponsible at best and, in my opinion, cause for an MD to lose their license at worst. Constipation for one day equates to not emptying the kitchen garbage can for a day. Continuing to eat and not eliminating is likened to continuing to throw garbage in an already full trash can and allowing it to pile up.

77

As constipation persists in the body, the trash can will begin to emit an odor as waste sits without a hope of disposal. The question as to why Americans develop gas, bloating, burping, heart burn and reflux is laughable. Is there really still someone out there who doesn't know the cause of these digestive issues? Are there really doctors who have gone to medical school for 10+ years who continue to prescribe harsh medications [which have recently shown a correlation to dementia (Gomm et al., 2016)] in an effort to get the body to do what it naturally knows how to do when fed real food?

If I sound upset, it's because I am! For goodness' sake, how many lions, bears, birds, or horses in the wild experience constipation? Is this a phenomenon specifically reserved for the human species or is it something we have created? The answer should be obvious.

If you are not eliminating at least twice a day, it is time to re-evaluate your body, your lifestyle, and of course, your diet. There is no "normal" for each person. We are part of a species and thus should function as the species functions. That is not to say that there won't be some slight variations based on each individual's level of stress, type of work, amount of exercise and/or volume of food consumed. However, if you eat what is natural to you as a species, it will be virtually impossible for you to not have at least two bowel movements a day. Preferably, one bowel movement after each meal. Please keep in mind that the elimination of waste should not have to be prompted, stimulated, or cajoled by coffee, laxatives, enemas, or even dietary supplements. Bowel movements should come easily and with no struggle just by virtue of your diet.

During detoxification, I always use an herbal formula to aid in bowel function. Whether you tend toward diarrhea, constipation, or anywhere in between, it is extremely important to support the digestive tract while on detox. The herbal formula is used not only to aid in the elimination of digestive and metabolic waste, but to support, clean and nourish the mucosa. "Mucosa" is another name for the mucus membrane that lines various cavities in the body, including the respiratory tract, and for the purposes of this chapter, the digestive tract. The mucosa secretes a thick protective fluid known as mucus, which helps to stop pathogens and dirt from entering the body. The innermost layer of the digestive tract, called the epithelium, is responsible for the secretion of mucus, allowing for digestion and absorption to occur. The use of the correct herbal formula in the proper dose will allow for optimal elimination without distress or the feeling of the body purging. It is important to state that these herbs are *only* used during the detoxification process and should not be needed or relied upon for elimination once detoxification is complete. That would amount to symptom treatment. As far as digestion, absorption, and elimination go, any issues should be corrected during detox. Once detox is over, a balanced whole food diet composed of a minimum of 80% alkaline foods will ensure that optimal elimination continues.

Healthy poop vs. unhealthy poop

So what do I mean by "healthy or unhealthy" poop? In traditional Chinese medicine, practitioners look at the body in great detail. We examine the skin, smell the breath, note every detail of the pulse, and inspect the tongue for color, shape, size, and coating. We ask many detailed questions regarding every function and system of the body. And yes, we ask about poop. How often does one have a bowel movement? Is there an urgency or sluggishness? Does bloating, gas, gurgling, or burping occur as part of digestion? What is the consistency of the stool? Is it loose, easily breaking apart? Is it hard, in small round balls, or long firm logs? Is it thin like a pencil? Does it float or sink? Is it gray, brown, black, or green? Finally, is undigested food present? These are all very important questions whose answers can aid in the choice of herbs, acupuncture points or gland tonics.

Is there a perfect poop? This is a question often asked in my office. The answer is yes and no. Perfect is a very precise term and because our diets stand to have an incredible amount of variation due to the vast variety or fruits and vegetables in the world, I will provide some basic characteristics of a healthy bowel movement.

- Firm but not hard.

- Soft but not watery or surrounded in mucus.

- There should be no blood.

- Stool should be eliminated in one or two long sections and should generally stay relatively "together" once passed (this can be quite different during detoxification).

- The color of the stool will tend to reflect the diet. Beets will turn the stool crimson, green juices will lead to greenish stool and sweet potatoes can make for a more orange elimination. Generally, stool should be medium to light brown and never gray or black.

- Clean up after one has a bowel movement should be easy and quick requiring a minimal amount of toilet paper and no other commercial "wipes."

- There should be no pain, bloating, or discomfort before or during elimination.

How to correct bowel issues

Whether the issue is diarrhea or constipation, improper eliminative habits must be corrected. As discussed throughout this book, I am not a fan of symptom treatment, nor the use of medication, vitamins, minerals, or long term use of herbs to prompt bowel movements, or slow them down. I strongly recommend detoxification to address and correct the root cause of digestive issues. Keep in mind that there are many prescription drugs as well as health issues (e.g. thyroid disease, adrenal weakness, neurological disorders) that can affect the body's ability to eliminate properly. On the flip-side, as stated earlier, poor elimination can lead to secondary health issues.

Here are just some health issues related to the digestive system:

- Irritable bowel syndrome (IBS)

- Colon cancer

- Diverticulitis/diverticulosis

- Colitis

- Crohn's disease

- Leaky gut

- Kidney stones

- Gall stones

- Diarrhea

- Constipation

When working to correct digestive issues with detoxification, one of the most important tools is iridology (see Chapter 14: "Recipes and resources"). Utilizing iridology allows the practitioner to get a clearer understanding of the digestive tract (as well as all other tissues of the body) so as to better determine the precise herbal protocol to use. This also allows the practitioner to incorporate adjunctive therapies into the detox process, such as acupuncture or cranial sacral therapy. In terms of a starting point when dealing with digestion problems, it is always advised to practice proper food-combining, as this can alleviate a multitude of digestive issues. While the appropriate herbs will serve to support the mucosa, proper food combining will ease digestion. Many secondary digestive organs such as the pancreas, gallbladder, and liver will have the opportunity to rest when food is ingested in a more simplistic manner. Consuming fruit as the first meal of the day is the best way to break-fast and ease the body back into the efforts of digestion. Fruit can be consumed throughout the morning, into the early afternoon, and for those who are really ready to dig deep in the detoxification process, fruit may be consumed into the evening as well. Whether you consume fruit up until mid-morning, lunch or afternoon, it is extremely important to note that *once you eat vegetables, do not go back to fruit for at least four hours.* This will ensure that the vegetables consumed will have a proper amount of time to be broken down and passed into the small intestine before fruit enters the body. This is the best and simplest way to avoid fermentation which leads to gas, bloating, flatulence, and belching. Proper food combining saves a great deal of money on Pepto-Bismol, Gas-X, Beeno, or probiotics!

Once gas, bloating, and the like are corrected, the issue of constipation can soon be a thing of the past. Fiber-rich fruits and vegetables will not only provide the proper medium for digestive waste to leave the body, but will also hydrate the bowels allowing for stool to bulk up and pass easily and cleanly. Conversely, many issues concerning diarrhea can also be corrected by adding fiber-rich foods which create a binding effect to the diet. Lastly, fruits and vegetables serve to scrub the walls of the colon, peeling away years of fatty foods and protein rich residue. To cleanse after long term consumption of processed foods containing grains, gluten, sugar, chemical colorants, and preservatives, a special herb and bentonite mixture is used to scrub the bowel walls deeply.

Many disorders of the bowels can be corrected by adding fiber to the diet in the form of live, raw fruits and vegetables. While a general rule of thumb in Western medicine is to limit or remove fiber from the diet of a colitis or Crohn's patient, the lack of fruit and vegetable fiber in the diet over a long period of time is a tremendous component in the cause of these disease processes. Of course, in a chronic condition, care must be taken when introducing high fiber into the diet of an IBS, Crohn's, or colitis patient. Along with detoxification and the proper herbs it is generally simple to bring about a positive change in these individuals. In the case of ulcerative colitis, the primary goal is to heal the ulcerations and stop bleeding in the intestines. Of course removing acids from the diet is enormously important, but in a case where the ulcerations are severe, one must stop all abrasive matter from coming in contact with the mucosa. Some practitioners use water fasting, and though I have not used this method myself, I know of cases where it has been incredibly successful. In my personal experience, blending a minimal number of fruits together in a smoothie or using a juicer to juice either fruits or vegetables is the best way to get a colitis patient on the road to recovery. I also love to use fresh coconut water. Living in South Florida allows me the opportunity to obtain fresh coconuts almost year round. Throughout these dietary changes I always use the appropriate herbs in the form of capsules, tinctures, and teas.

A word about the sexes

It is not uncommon to see trends in digestion in the sexes. I often field questions from female patients regarding obvious differences from their male counterparts when it comes to bathroom habits. Although they share the same diet, the women may have a great deal of trouble with constipation while their husbands "go like clockwork." To this I say, s**t happens! Seriously, I have no idea why this occurs but I can offer a few things to consider:

1. Amount of water consumed.

2. Amount of physical activity or exercise.

3. Amount of downtime (often women are in rush-mode and don't allow enough time to just "sit" in the bathroom). In a hectic lifestyle, if you don't stop to go when you feel the urge, you may lose the moment.

4. Consumption of coffee or other stimulants. Not that I recommend coffee or energy drinks, but it is possible that your significant other may be consuming these products which can cause a strong stimulant effect on the nervous system as well as digestion. Often when one stops consuming these products during detox, even with a huge increase of natural dietary fiber, bowel movements slow down and constipation can occur (herein lies another reason for the appropriate herbal formula).

5. Hormonal factors, especially in a woman who is still menstruating, can affect elimination as well.

While I tend to see constipation more often in women than in their male counterparts it is certainly not limited to women. For various reasons including diet, men can experience constipation as well. These specific issues are addressed on an individual basis in regard to herbs and other GI cleansers.

"A day without sunshine is like, you know, night."

- Steve Martin

C | U | R | E *quotes*

Chapter 7
Duh!!!

My husband would probably say this is an obnoxious title for a chapter in a book. Especially a book that takes a serious look at the human health condition, causes of illness and disease, and their resolution (C.U.R.E.). But for me, humor is a very powerful and necessary tool in the process of healing the body. Therefore, this chapter contains just some of the countless thoughts that find their way in and out of the crevices of my brain which cause me to say "Duh, that's why it's... (Fill in the blank)!"

There are so many books, websites, blogs, and such at our disposal these days, each touting the *"real answer"* to how you should eat, take care of your health, and prevent or reverse disease. Numerous plausible and implausible theories abound, from eating according to your blood type, to hypothesizing what our ancient ancestors ate, to choosing one macronutrient (protein) as the poster child of all nutrients. It is confusing to say the least, while frustrating and difficult to follow at best. As I mentioned in Chapter 1, my husband and I have been vegan for 24+ years and we are frequently barraged with questions regarding our dietary choices.

On most occasions we answer questions about our diet thoughtfully, with our own life experiences in mind, while other times we refer to strong, science-based evidence. Then there are those moments when we want to clunk someone in the head (much like the old V8 commercial) and say "Duh...!" That *duh* moment is the inspiration for this chapter. It begs you to look at life simplistically, not as a scientist or researcher. Not as someone searching for an award or for recognition that their (current) health or nutrition theory is *the* truth of the decade. That *duh* moment that makes you realize that all of the

intellect in the world cannot compete with the information your own body tells you EVERY DAY!

Duh #1: Our anatomy dictates our natural diet.

It will come as no shock to you that I believe humans should subsist on a primarily plant based diet. But which *duh* moment brought me to this conclusion? The answer lies in simple anatomy.

When a paleontologist unearths the bones of an ancient species, scientist scramble to understand everything about it that they possibly can. Where did it live, was it nomadic, what was the range of size within the species; did it have skin, fur, or scales and what did it eat? All of these questions can be answered just by studying the anatomy of the creature.

Bones and teeth are all that is left of the animal when it is unearthed thousands and thousands of years after its demise. Yet, by analyzing these basic and foundational parts, scientists can come to reasonably accurate conclusions about an animal's life. Comparatively speaking however, we seem to ignore our own anatomy and what it is screaming at us about our nature and our diet.

If we look at the basics, it is evident that a high (animal) protein diet is not what our anatomy dictates we consume. First of all, let's analyze what we can see clearly. You know what I am talking about, the thing that catches your eye when you first meet someone. Yes, your smile! Or more specifically, your teeth! Your teeth are the most powerful and clear indicators of what the human species is meant to eat (duh moment). For those of you who feel that we are carnivores, I ask you this… If I let a live rabbit loose in a field, are you able to drop down to the ground, run around on all fours, catch the rabbit with just your mouth and teeth, shake it until its neck snaps and then proceed to eat it without cooking it?

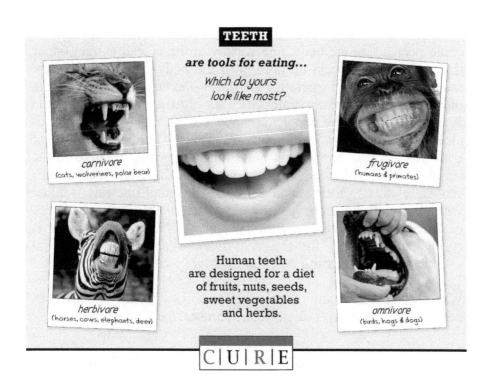

TEETH

are tools for eating...
Which do yours
look like most?

carnivore
(cats, wolverines, polar bear)

frugivore
(humans & primates)

Human teeth
are designed for a diet
of fruits, nuts, seeds,
sweet vegetables
and herbs.

herbivore
(horses, cows, elephants, deer)

omnivore
(birds, hogs & dogs)

C | U | R | E

I must strongly argue against the concept that the human species is carnivorous! (Please see the chart below that depicts the teeth of different species, including that of a carnivore). I don't suspect you will do well either, down on your hands and knees with your head dropped between your arms, grazing on some thick, fibrous grass. Keep in mind that we are using our eyes and exploring anatomy right now. We are not discussing the invention of tools or the harnessing of fire.

The fact is that your teeth are very well suited for the consumption of fruit, vegetables, (as long as they are not too fibrous like grasses), and small amounts of nuts or seeds. If you are not detoxifying or do not have a health issue (e.g. headaches, fatigue, menstrual issues, autoimmune disorders, fertility issues, or cancer) you can consume a small amount of animal protein (free range, organic, grass fed, antibiotic-free) which amounts to no more than a chimpanzee would consume (3–4% of its total diet) or around what a silver-back gorilla would consume (1–2% of its diet). This is clearly what your teeth dictate you eat.

Putting on our x-ray vision glasses, let's look a little deeper. If we could peer inside the body, specifically at the digestive tract (since this is the food processing portion of the body) we would see the interior of the mouth (secreting amylase—the enzyme which aids in the digestion of carbohydrates such as glucose in vegetation and fructose in fruit), the esophagus, and an intestinal tract that was clearly designed to process plants and fruits. The digestive tract of both humans and primates is quite long, especially relative to the length of the spinal column. In carnivores, the digestive tract is much shorter relative to their spinal column. The small intestine is filled with micro-villi which have one main focus, to absorb the vast array of micronutrients found in fruits and plants. The large intestine is corrugated, allowing for the vital task of absorbing water and vitamins while converting digested food into feces.

When all is said and done, the anatomy speaks volumes in determining our species' diet. In one phrase, "the EYES have it!"

Duh #2: Toilet paper speak volumes about our natural diet.

Toilet paper. It's a great invention. As far as I know, the general design concept of toilet paper has not changed for, well, forever.

My *duh moment* came when I was about two weeks into detox. Of course, I was experiencing many changes in my body. Some of those transformations were wonderful, like the slowing of my extremely elevated heart rate due to thyroid disease, while others were not so wonderful, like a pounding headache which lingered for five days. This *duh moment* occurred when I was finishing up my "business" in the bathroom. The toilet paper roll was down to the last few squares (and for the Seinfeld fans, since I was alone at home, there was no one to ask if they could "spare a square") so I was concerned, knowing that I always use more than just a few squares for an average um…clean up. Since I did not have a backup roll in the bathroom vanity, I decided to do my best with what I had and then duck-walk to the garage for more TP. What happened next really made me think. Without getting into too much detail, I realized that just a few squares was all I needed! And, I probably could have used less than that! There was virtually no "residue" on the paper after the wipe!

I wondered, how could this be? I began to ponder the question of TP in a very simplistic way. Do humans use toilet paper because we are more sophisticated or more evolved than other species? Or is it possible that we have gotten so far away from our natural diet and what our species should eat that our waste has become a very sticky, messy, and well, toxic affair? While sitting there, thoughts arose and I began to envision other species and their elimination process. My horse, cat, or dog; a wild bird flying overhead, sharks, elephants— the list went on and on, and yet I could not think of any animal species that had to clean itself after defecating.

As you watch television (and I hope you don't do that too often) with its numerous commercials advertising stronger, sturdier, and softer toilet paper or new adult moist wipes, it is evident that cleaning ourselves is becoming a more and more labor and tool intensive process. And as always, my question is *why?*

After eating a pure fruit and vegetable detox diet, it became clear to me that if you eat what is natural to your species, you can eliminate waste with hardly any necessity for a cleanup crew! However, if you consume a typical American diet filled with high protein, mucus-forming dairy, and glue-like grains, well, your process of elimination and cleanup will be a sticky, pasty, gluey, and tacky mess! *Duh!* If you don't believe me, just give a clean diet a try for a few weeks.

Duh #3: Babies are the key to how often humans should eliminate.

As a practitioner of acupuncture, I ask many detailed questions about a patient's body. One of the most common remarks my new patients make is, "Wow, you ask more questions than any other doctor I have ever seen." In addition to a six page questionnaire, I spend at least 60 minutes out of a 90 minute consultation with each new patient gathering as much information as possible. Several of my questions focus on digestion and bowel habits (yes, it IS a crappy conversation, but someone has to have it!). There are the expected queries regarding heart burn, reflux, bloating, and gas. But then I dig deeper, looking to understand how often they have a bowel movement and how it appears—volume, shape, color, and whether there is any undigested food present. It never ceases to amaze me how many people (often women) tell me that they have a bowel movement every two, three, four days, or even longer! When I ask if they think that is acceptable, they usually reply "Well, I asked my doctor and they said that this is *normal for me.*"

Is there a "normal for me?" Again, looking toward simplicity, I ponder the bowel habits of a baby. Newborns, several weeks old, or several months old, it doesn't matter. Just think about how often a baby has a bowel movement. Often it is within moments or up to 20 minutes after a meal. It can happen again before the next meal and certainly after each meal of the day. The more they eat, the more they poop.

Yet babies are not eliminating what they just ate. It is the act of eating (more so, chewing and swallowing) that triggers the autonomic nervous system response known as peristalsis. Peristalsis is the same thing that causes those noises that you hear in your abdomen after a meal. It is a wonderful thing, transporting each morsel of food from the moment we swallow to the stomach (for chemical as well as mechanical digestion), then into the small intestine (for absorption of nutrients) and finally, digestive waste is moved into the large intestine until it reaches the end of the line for elimination. Without peristalsis, digestive waste would just continue to build up in the colon and you wouldn't have a bowel movement multiple times a day. Or once a day. Or every other day. You see, peristalsis and multiple daily bowel movements ARE NORMAL! Anything less is just abnormal, wrong, and against the nature of our species. So why would your doctor say it is "normal for you?" Better yet, why would you or your doctor believe that once you reach a certain age, multiple daily bowel movements are not normal or necessary for you? Common sense dictates otherwise. *Typical function should not be misconstrued for normal function.*

The other part of that equation is the stool's consistency. Hard, small, round balls? Long and skinny? Thick and short? Sticky or gooey? This is covered in more detail in Chapter 6: "The Process of

Elimination."

So how do you achieve multiple daily bowel movements of significant size, volume, and consistency? Eat what is natural to our species. What is that? A plant-based diet of course! Lots of fruits and vegetables (please refer to "Duh #1: Shouldn't it be clear what the human species should eat?"). Look to babies as your *duh moment* when it comes to how often you should eliminate.

Duh #4: Babies–the key to our desire for fruit.

"Fruit has too much sugar. I don't eat fruit because it is not good to eat all of that sugar." This is the second most popular statement I hear whenever I am asked about my diet or the detoxification diet (the #1 statement is found in Chapter 4). The extraordinary fear of fruit that has developed in this country conjures up scenes from the classic movie *"Attack of the Killer Tomatoes."* As wickedly giant tomatoes (which are, in fact, fruit) roll around the city attacking unsuspecting citizens, screams and mayhem break out! I am faced with similar bouts of panic when I instruct patients to eat as much fruit as they can.

As we look back to Duh #1, we can understand by means of our anatomy that plants, especially fruits, are the most natural foods a human can eat. However, the concern of fruit sugar, or fructose, began to take hold of the population when Dr. Atkins first introduced his book, *Dr. Atkins' Diet Revolution*. The push for high protein foods and the removal of all carbs, including fruit, set off a chain reaction in the American culture causing many of them to virtually boycott nature's perfect food. (Side note: Americans are fatter and sicker than they ever were pre-Atkins; and Atkins is deceased with all of his high protein attributes).

Although fruit and its energy-producing sugar, fructose get a bum rap from weight loss experts and nutritional authorities, the gurus of food (babies and children) prevail and have given me that *duh moment*. As they say, "out of the mouths of babes." For our purposes it is more like "into the mouth of babes!" As we observe the human as a species, we see that human babies LOVE fruit. When given the choice (fruit, veggies, or animal flesh) they will virtually always choose fruit. This is of course provided that their taste buds were not contaminated with processed food. Is this because babies are addicted to sugar? NO! A four, six, or eight month old baby is not addicted to sugar. Addiction to fruit sugar would be likened to someone having an addiction to water or air! You need these elements to live, but that does not make it an addiction.

Now if you are referring to the sugar that is in Cheerios, that is a totally different story. They may not add a great deal of sugar to that common breakfast treat, but maltose is the natural sugar occurring in all grains and, news flash, grains are highly addictive! I cannot truly visualize a baby sitting in its high chair with a bowl of fresh cut watermelon unable to stop eating, but I sure have seen little ones pile drive Cheerios or Goldfish crackers until all that remains are artificially colored orange crumbs! That is a sugar craving that you just can't turn off. The more you eat, the more you want.

As an adult that may be struggling with their weight, if you had a magic wand to take you back in time and stop you from eating that first bite of cereal, slice of bread, or bowl of pasta, would you not be waving it right now like a maniac? Would you agree that it is virtually impossible to avoid that second bowl of pasta or second slice of bread and butter? But, would you really wish that you never had that first bite of banana, juicy peach, or succulent melon? Does eating fruit feel like an addiction or like a cool, sweet, hydrating bath for every cell of your body? Can I hear a *DUH???*

Duh #5: Micro-nutrients determine hunger and the body's need for food, not feeling "full." Just counting protein, fat, carbs, points or calories does not give the body what it needs nutritionally. This kind of mathematics gives us a false sense of nutritional security.

The American Diabetic Association looks very closely at the glycemic index when guiding a diabetic patient's diet. The focus remains on how a carbohydrate-containing food raises the blood sugar and oftentimes ignores the complete nutrient profile of the food. I once listened to a nurse tell her patient that a brownie and a white potato are equal on the glycemic index and therefore it makes no difference which one the person chooses as long as they are looking at the total number of glucose points for the day. If you follow this logic you will find that diabetics tend to remain diabetic and hungry!

The same holds true for weight loss diets, especially those that follow some kind of calorie counting system or point scheme. These programs may work for a while but ultimately the participant in this type of diet will feel hungry and deprived, resulting in "falling off the wagon." I know what you are thinking. "Doesn't a detox diet *deprive* me of the foods I want?" The answer to that lies here in Duh #5.

Hunger is based on the body getting what it needs, not what the mind wants. What I mean by this is, if you flood the body with real, live, nutritious food containing all of the essential amino acids, sugars, and fats, as well as the vitamins and minerals it requires, you would find that body fat easily balances to a natural weight, blood sugar completely normalizes, and best of all, cravings disappear! Why? Because hunger and cravings are not based on the lack of points, calories, proteins, or sugars in the diet. Nor is it based on an empty organ known as the stomach. It is based on cells getting what they need to function optimally. If you give your body and your taste buds the opportunity to reacquaint themselves with the delicious taste sensations of REAL FOOD, you will discover two very important things:

1. Detoxification is much easier than you thought.

2. It will be incredibly painless to eat a healthy and natural diet once the detoxification process is complete.

If you are not sure, just try it. You are your own scientist. Besides, you remember the definition of insanity, don't you? *The act of doing the same thing over and over and expecting a different result.* How many times have you or someone you know embarked on a weight loss program? In all of your years on this planet, have you seen the weight of Americans as a whole increase or decrease? Has the American Medical Association won the war on diabetes, heart disease, high blood pressure, autoimmune diseases, or cancer? Or *anything?* The doctors and scientists that tell you that vaccines do not cause autism are the same doctors and scientists that told me Graves' disease is incurable. You do the math. Eat a clean, living diet and see how content and full you will feel, not to mention how you will reverse the process of disease in your body and C.U.R.E. what ails you.

Duh #6: Maintaining optimal weight is not a science, it is a product of nature.

This duh moment is very much connected to duh #5. Although this book is not about weight loss, a very common side effect of detoxification is almost always the loss of weight. As much as I feel for the person who has spent their life bouncing from one weight loss scheme to another, I am angered by the establishment (you know who they are…the drug companies, protein shake, supplement, exercise video, 100 calorie snack, and medical industries that continue to sell their products under the guise of giving a damn about people!) who arguably knows the truth but continues to play the public. They try to convince us that obesity is a malfunction of the brain and how it interprets hunger. They plead their case that obesity is a diagnosable disease. They work the angle that we overeat due to an emotional disorder. Though there are certainly instances where disease and emotional issues are directly related to over (or under) eating, the fact is that the vast majority of overweight or obese individuals are a product of industry turning humans against their nature. The food, pharmaceutical, and medical industries want us to believe that there is a hidden cause for obesity lurking just around the corner. Apparently, the next fad diet, fat-burning and appetite suppressing pill, or radical surgical procedure will be the answer to our obesity woes. But what they fail to disclose is that the industrialization of food and the mass production of processed foods, sugar-free treats, low-calorie this and low-fat that drives Americans deeper and deeper into a hole that they struggle to get out of.

This mass brain washing starts earlier and earlier with each generation. Just look at the garbage they serve in school that is supposed to nourish our children at the peak of their growth and brains' development. Theories on nutrition get transferred from industry, to the government, and finally to the public in the form of the ever changing food pyramid. A "balanced" eating program designed by industry, not science, in an effort to sell more commodities and make greater profits, all while digging a larger and larger hole for our caskets is not what we should rely upon for nutritional advice. If I sound pissed, I am! (Just look at the title of this chapter!) If you believe the pyramid was designed by the greatest scientists and nutritionists our nation could muster, think again!

White sugar is not food! Processed grains are not food! Milk from another species is not food! Moreover, dead animal flesh on your plate 2–3 times a day serves only to make you sicker and the industry's bank accounts fatter! Yes, the food, drug, and medical industries all profit greatly from the effects this ridiculous pyramid has on your diet. Let's look at this logically…

How often do you see an overweight humming bird? When do you ever catch an otter "pinching an inch" of his waist? When you donate to "save the whales," do you think that means save them because they are fat (whales) and need a diet? Do you get my point? There is no animal that exists in nature who is overweight! All animals maintain optimal weights (though in cases of drought or famine they may be underweight) by eating what is natural to their species! Please say it with me…DUH!!!

When we turn back to nature and take time to understand what a natural diet is for the human species, we find that it is nearly impossible to be overweight! Even if you are not detoxifying, eating a natural human diet will make you feel incredible. The necessity to count calories and points, Zumba yourself to exhaustion, kill your appetite with dangerous pills, or have parts of your God-given digestive tract removed or strangled (via bariatric surgery and lap bands) will seem so exceedingly absurd that you will never go there again.

Weight loss is not a science and does not require scientific breakthroughs in order to be accomplished. Maintaining an optimal weight should be attainable if you detoxify your body and eat what is natural to the human species. We will discuss how to move forward with your diet after you have detoxified in Chapter 14: "Recipes & resources."

Duh #7: Seasonal depression disorder proves that human's true nature is to live in the tropics.

Can you survive naked outdoors, all year long, in the part of the world which you currently reside (barring arrest of course)? Even though our intellect has allowed us to figure out how to overcome the obstacle of frigid weather, it is plainly obvious that we are not naturally suited to live in those conditions. Freezing weather is not suitable for providing fresh fruit and vegetation found in the tropics and sub-tropics. These foods flourished in Southern Ethiopia where it is believed the crucible of human life began (the 2.8 million year old genus homo species).

We have wandered from end to end of the globe for various reasons, including an insatiable desire to know more about our world. Yet, the effort it takes for us to survive and sustain ourselves in these regions, from food to clothing to heat to artificial sunlight makes it clear to me that a tropical region is much more our nature then Seattle, Canada, or the Antarctic. I have nothing against these areas or the people who live there, but the correlation between a natural place for us to live and a natural diet must be drawn. An easy way to do so is to understand the profound effect the lack of sustained sunlight has on our body, mind, and emotions.

From a holistic point of view, if the lack of sustained sunlight can cause us to feel sad, depressed, or have a weakened immune system, then it stands to reason (holistically) that the other aspects that go along with that environment (water, temperature, and food) must be vitally important to our survival as well. The industry would like you to believe that you are just lacking a vitamin D pill, and once you buy the latest and greatest formulation of that pill, all will be well. Oh yes, I know there are people who live in the sunshine state of Florida who are low in vitamin D even when most days are sunny and bright. There are various reasons for a vitamin D deficiency, some of which have nothing to do with sunlight, but that does not preclude that fact that sunshine is staple of human life.

Technological interventions are helpful in the fight against seasonal depression if you live in a less than optimal environment, but there is no substitute for sunshine and the variety of natural foods this climate fosters.

Duh #8: Stop relying on nutritionists, doctors, bodybuilders, and the government to determine human protein requirements and put your faith in your mother! If you really want to understand how much (or how little) protein humans need, look at breast milk! Duh!!!

The topic of protein during and after detoxification is covered in great detail during Chapter 4: "Where do you get your protein?" But for the *Duh* chapter, I wanted the explanation of human protein needs to be concise and simple. Today there are numerous points of view regarding how much protein we should consume in a day. This is often followed by opinions on the optimal source of protein for the human species.

These opinions tend to be regurgitated citations of exercise and sports professionals, nutritionists, or the ever popular US Food Pyramid. I have even heard of research performed on other mammals, such as rats (Osborn and Mendel; 1914), to determine what combinations of amino acids (the building blocks of protein) are just right for a human. There are so many individuals who consider themselves authorities on the topic, it could make your head spin. But, when I research information regarding any of our nutritional needs, I like to go to the source.

In the case of protein, my source of information rests in something my mom once told me, "Mothers know everything!" And you know, she was right. Mothers hold the final word when it comes to nutrition for their babies. If we simply follow their logic as we mature, it should be quite easy to determine just how much protein we require for optimal health.

For decades, sports heroes, paid actors, and "revolutionary" doctor/authors have persuaded us to believe that high protein was the answer to our obesity, diabetic, and cholesterol woes. Once the corporate American food industry caught wind of the protein revolution, there was virtually no stopping it! Americans happily jumped on the bandwagon of endless sausage, steak, and bacon! But where did these so-called "experts" get their information? What study, research, or lab experiment lead them to their protein conclusions?

I realized that science almost exclusively uses Mickey Mouse's cousin to determine all sorts of facts, figures, and data for humans. Rats can help scientists conclude which drugs might kill us vs. which drugs may only maim us. But studying this mid-size rodent to determine the nutritional requirements of humans is just, well, Goofy! However, if we use a little common sense and query the most intelligent beings on the planet, as to how much protein a human requires, they would give us the right answer 100% of the time. Who are these gurus of nutrition? Moms of course! Let me explain.

Breast milk is the first food of all mammals on the planet, specifically provided by the mother of the species. It is the perfect food to nourish an infant from birth (which grows, supports, and develops them) to a point where they can eat on their own. Breast milk provides not only sustenance for a baby but a vast amount of information for science in regards to the nutritional needs of over 5,500 mammals on the planet.

But somehow science took a different direction. They concluded that the best way to determine the nutritional needs of a *baby, toddler, teen, or adult* is to define what foods would allow a *rat* to grow and thrive and then to analyze those foods for their amino acid content. Based on those components, scientists would define the protein needs of a human. Makes sense, right? WRONG! This not only stares sense in the face and spits in it, this line of reasoning borders on conspiracy. You knew I would use the word conspiracy eventually, didn't you? Yes, I had to go there! But after all, who stands to gain in this protein revolution? You or the corporations selling millions of dollars' worth of books and magazines as well as protein shakes, bars, powders, and enriched food-like products?

So, let's observe nature's perfect food. Of the 5,500+ mammals who produce and feed their young breast milk, human breast milk contains the lowest amount of protein of any species (*Roy et al., 1990*).

Casein, the protein portion of all milk, is species-specific. This means that in various species, the amino acid composition of casein is vastly different, specifically meeting the needs of the offspring of the species who produce it. What also varies greatly is the ratio of casein to whey. Human breast milk has the lowest ratio of casein to whey of any species of mammal. You may ask why the amount of protein in breast milk is important. There are several reasons.

1. Protein serves the purpose of developing skeletal muscle at a rapid rate. This allows an animal to be able to locomote at a very young age, providing protection from predators.

2. Early human development, unlike other mammals', is dependent upon the consumption of fat for the benefit of the brain and nervous system. The human neurological system is not fully developed at birth and since brain matter (and Schwan cells which cover nerves) is largely made of fatty tissue, a high protein milk will hinder brain development. Cow milk for example is geared for muscular development, not brain development.

3. High protein milk will increase a baby's body weight rapidly but will have a negative impact on brain tissue. Data shows that children raised on cow milk, on average, have a lower IQ than children raised on human breast milk. *(Dr. Walter J. Veith — "Udderly Amazing")*

Let's take a look at the amount of protein in the milks of various species as well as the time required for an infant to double its birth weight. *(please see chart on the following page)*

Growth Chart

	Mean value for protein content of breast milk	Time required to double birth weight
	mg/liter	days
Human	1.2	120
Horse	2.4	60
Cow	3.3	47
Goat	4.1	19
Dog	7.1	8
Cat	9.5	7
Rat	11.8	4.5

C | U | R | E

If you are looking for milk with the highest source of protein, look no more. Yes, rat milk will provide you will all the excess protein your fitness trainer or fat-burning weight loss book could ask for. All at the expense of your wonderful kidneys. You remember your kidneys from Chapter 2: "The Science of Sickness?" The kidneys are bestowed with the responsibility of removing cellular waste, including the waste products of protein metabolism (ammonia, urea, and uric acid). And just like any organ, tissue, or gland of the body, they have a max capacity at which they can operate. Asking the kidneys to work above their max capacity every now and then is certainly possible and as Americans, we do it every day. But when those days turn into weeks, months, years or decades, kidney function will steadily decline making kidney disease one of the fastest growing health epidemics in modern society. The Journal of the American Medical Association found that 13 percent of American adults (about 26 million people) have chronic kidney disease (CKD), up from 10 percent (or about 20 million people), a decade earlier. The amount of adults aged 30 or older who have CKD is projected to increase from 13.2% currently, to 14.4% in

2020 and 16.7% in 2030. While there are certainly chemical components that contribute to kidney disease (such as toxins in our household, countless jobs where chemical exposure is a norm, drugs, excessive alcohol consumption and processed food), Americans' insatiable appetites for high protein diets is the most prevalent causative factor in modern society. Other disease processes such as diabetes and vascular disease (which are also a product of high protein) are primary diseases that can eventually lead to CKD. So, when the next magazine advertisement asks if you *"got milk?"* or your trainer pushes you to increase your protein intake, you may want to refer back to good old mom. The amount of protein she provided for you to double your birth weight in just 120 days is vastly lower than the protein content in all other mammals' milk. What any of the "experts" dictate regarding how much protein is necessary for adult health and fitness is likely more suitable for your dog than for you.

Corporate America's greed has led to an obsession with protein, propelling Americans down a rabbit hole of lies and inconsistencies. We follow the follower, repeating the same misinformation about humans' nutritional needs from the latest fitness magazine or weight loss craze our best friend quoted just last week. The result is an extraordinarily negative impact on our state of health, including rampant disease, epidemic obesity, and increasing issues of cognition in both the young and elderly.

So what about protein needs of children, teens and adults? Once we are weaned from the breast and move to solid food, do our protein needs significantly change? In adulthood, the type of protein the human species needs *does not change!* We are not suddenly able to digest cow milk. We do not develop the need to put on excessive muscle tissue (sorry, Arnold!) at the risk of our brain, nervous system, immune system, or bones. We do not grow fangs and require more flesh over fruit. An adult elephant eats the same plants a baby elephant eats. A young lion eats the same dead animal flesh his older siblings and parents eat. A full grown man who runs, lifts weights, and participates in obstacle course races (see Chapter 4: "Where do you get your protein?" and take note of the photo) still eats what his young niece or nephew eats. It stands to reason that our caloric intake increases as we grow and expend more energy, but the nutrient ratios in our food remains the same.

Choosing your food based on the nutritional needs of a rat or the latest weight-loss craze *makes no sense!* Say it with me…*DUH!!!*

Duh #9: While we are on the subject of dairy and human health, let's set things straight once and for all. Just because you "like" to consume something, doesn't mean you should! Duh!

There are many edible, drinkable, and inhalable "natural" substances in the world that man has experimented with, only to find that they lead to his demise. But none are more socially acceptable than dairy. On a nutritional basis, milk and all of its offspring have single handedly brought about human suffering so great that the only thing more powerful than the havoc it wreaks on our bodies is our addiction to it.

There are literally thousands of products on the market containing milk or some component of milk like casein, whey, lactose, or galactose. From gallons of this liquid poison to soft and hard cheeses, yogurt, and ice cream to margarine, canned tuna, dairy-free cheese, non-dairy coffee creamer, semisweet chocolate, cereal bars, cheese-flavored chips and snack crackers, processed meats, ghee, baked goods, infant formulas, breath mints, glaze for baked goods, salad dressings, processed meats, cereals, protein powders, nutrition bars, and any foods with whipped toppings. Whew! That's a lot of stuff. Milk is one of the most processed foods on the planet. And speaking of the planet, the raising of dairy cows for the consumption of their milk (and subsequent flesh for ground beef) is one of the most resource-depleting processes humans have ever created. Water use, land use, and cow excrement causes so much harm to this planet that it would take an entire book to address this issue (please refer to "Diet for a New America" in the resource section for more information).

For now, let's focus on dairy's harm to the human body. In his lecture "*Udderly amazing*," Dr. Walter J. Veith addresses many of the health issues directly connected to the consumption of cow milk. Much of the issues are due to casein (milk protein) and galactose (milk sugar which the human digestive system has great difficulty digesting). These are just a few:

1. 30% increased risk of intestinal bleeding leading to iron loss in the stool of babies 6 months and older (Journal of Pediatrics, 1992)

2. Adults who have consumed milk and dairy products throughout their lives have a greater likelihood in developing senile cataracts (Postgraduate Medicine, 1994)

3. Increases cholesterol (Journal of Dairy Science, 1991)

4. Iron deficiency syndrome

5. Type I diabetes (American Journal of Clinical Nutrition 1990; New England Journal of Medicine, 1992)

6. Ovarian cancer (Lancet, 1989)

7. Infertility

8. Osteoporosis (American Journal of Clinical Nutrition, 1974)

9. Allergies

10. Asthma

11. Eczema

12. Toxins such as pesticides and antibiotics

There is no doubt Americans are addicted to their dairy and we are pushing our insatiable habit onto other countries around the world. This will continue to lead to environmental destruction and the deterioration of our health. From a detoxification standpoint, dairy is the #1 food product to be removed from the human diet. If it is not removed, detoxification will not occur. So, true or false..." milk does a body good?" FALSE! Duh!

Duh #10: I get massive headaches when I stop drinking coffee, so maybe I should not stop?

Inevitably, sometime in my workweek, one of my patients will tell me about a study they read touting the health benefits of coffee. The beneficial claims range from preventing diabetes and lowering the incidence of Parkinson's disease, to protecting against heart failure and increasing antioxidant levels in the body. If you conduct a Google search, you can find these same health benefits from the leaf of the coca (cocaine) plant. You may be hard pressed to choose whether cocaine or coffee is more addictive.

Much like quitting cigarettes, illicit drugs, or alcohol can yield a laundry list of uncomfortable withdrawal side effects, the cessation of caffeine consumption can also produce withdrawal symptoms. When we remove stimulants from the body that we have grown accustomed to for months, years, or even decades, the body goes into withdrawal. The desire for these products can become overwhelming and if enough time has passed (12–48 hours) since their cessation, the body will begin to purge (detox) the lingering chemistry left behind from years of use. The purging of toxic chemistry can lead to headaches, skin rashes, sweating, nausea, and several other uncomfortable symptoms.

Should you therefore forego the discomfort and keep coffee in your system? The answer will be the same whether we are talking about caffeine, cigarettes, or cocaine...NO! DUH! Just because a food or food product has some beneficial health component in it does not mean it is a health food and should be consumed on a regular basis. You can find all the benefits of coffee in thousands of fresh fruits and vegetables that do not contain stimulants. The act of stimulating your adrenal glands (via a fight or flight response) to squeeze out that last little bit of adrenaline to wake you up in the morning or get you through your afternoon lull at work is not real energy. I could accomplish the same thing by holding a gun to your head at 5:45 a.m. as a way to *encourage* you to get out of bed and start your day. The threat of a gun at your temple stimulates the same adrenal response of fight or flight, which will absolutely prompt your movement to start your day. But is it a good, healthy, or natural way to get you going in the morning? Neither is coffee.

Now I know what you are going to say. Yes, having a cup of coffee to wake you up in the morning is a far cry from the threat of a gun. And you are right. But that cup of coffee usually does not stop at one. There is the second and sometimes third morning cup, then the afternoon pick-me-up followed by the evening "energy" drink at the gym. Not to mention the fact that coffee is consumed year after year on a daily basis by most people. Anything that you "need" in order to get going, which causes mild to extreme symptoms if you stop its consumption, must be eliminated from the diet during detox and reduced significantly after detox. Oftentimes, my patients who have consumed coffee prior to detox ask if they can resume drinking it once the detoxification process is over. Since I agree that a little bit of coffee, chocolate, or wine can certainly be tolerated by the body, I encourage them to experiment. Usually a half cup of coffee after 16 weeks of detox will speak for itself. Jitteriness, elevated heart rate, and sleep disturbance are a few of the effects of coffee in a newly cleansed body! Many patients choose to discontinue it completely, while others like my husband will have it as a "treat" once or twice a week. At that rate, the body will not become addicted to it, adrenal glands won't have the life squeezed out of them and they can actually learn to truly appreciate the taste and feeling of a good, hot, and rich cup of coffee.

Duh #11: Does it make sense that humans are allergic to their environment (seasonal allergies; dust; mold etc.)? Do animals in the wild have environmental allergies?

Allergies are one of my favorite topics, mostly because I don't really believe in them. "You don't believe in allergies?!" many of my patients ask skeptically. No, I really don't. At least not for the majority of allergens. Seriously, how can I believe in something that I can make disappear in most cases, without any drugs, allergy shots, or hypo-allergenic redecoration of the home (special beds, pillows, carpet etc.)? I don't believe in allergies because I don't believe that the human species can innately be allergic to its natural environment—the great outdoors! How often do you hear of a lion, tiger, or bear having allergies?

How far removed have we become from nature that we cannot come in contact with it for fear of sneezing, itching, or rashes? Why do our eyes water around our pets and mucus congests our lungs when we blow the feathery petals of a dandelion? Is it because we were born with a part of our body that hyper-reacts to the environment for no known reason? Is it because our parents were allergic to cats so we will be as well? Is it because…hmmm, because…because…we don't even know why! After 10 years of med-school, umpteen years in a medical practice and countless "scientific studies," not even modern medicine can explain why we get allergies. Maybe we are just looking at this issue from the wrong point of view, the point of view that treats symptoms (for lots of money mind you) and is not really interested in the cause.

For a greater description of cause, please refer back to Chapter 2, "The Science of Sickness." For now, allow me to give you a visual. Pretend that you have an empty 50 gallon drum sitting by your front door. Every time you walk through the door, I would like you to use an eye dropper and squeeze one drop of milk into the drum. Each time you leave the house for work, to meet a friend, get the mail, walk the dog, or receive a delivery you will squeeze a drop of milk into the drum. Furthermore, every time you return home, you will squeeze another drop of milk into the drum. At first you might look at the drum and wonder how it will ever fill up. But at some point it will be clear that the drops do, in fact, add up. The next thing you should notice is that the milk becomes rancid. It curdles, turning thick as its texture changes. Finally one day, years down the road, you squeeze just one more drop into the 50 gallon drum and it overflows. Just one drop at a time over the period of many years willeventually fill up the drum until it reaches capacity and overflows! Not to mention the utterly horrid stench that emanates from it.

This is basically what happens in the human body, sometimes slowly over decades while other times quite rapidly over several months. It is all based on how many (acidic) drops you put into your vessel at a time. Today, children are weaned on acid. They are quickly taken away from their mother's breast (if they were even given it at all) and fed a scientifically "balanced" mixture of laboratory created pre-digested proteins, chemicals, grains, and sugars. This "nutrition" is designed to feed a rapidly growing and neurologically developing body. The only thing this swill is developing is an over acidic, congesting, and putrefying 50 gallon drum! Allowing the body to build such a horrific internal environment of non-foods and unnatural substances creates a situation where contact with the natural environment will stimulate a reaction. Why? Because a lymphatically congested nasal passage, sinus cavity, throat, tonsil (provided they have not been butchered out of the body), or lung is not viscous enough to allow dust, pollen, and dander to enter and be easily moved through the system which eventually eliminates it through the kidneys, colon, or skin (again, Chapter 2). Instead, natural substances like tree pollen become trapped in the cesspool of dirty lymph, creating thick mucus and an "allergic-like" response. Clean up the cesspool by eliminating the congesting, acidic culprits and the allergies magically go away! No drugs or years of allergy shots required. No removal of body parts such as adenoids or tonsils necessary. No home redecorating needed. Just pure alkalization. After all, how can you feed living cells dead food and expect those cells to function properly?

I know it is challenging these days to prepare food for yourself, your significant other, and your child. But what choices do you have? Are you comfortable putting your five-year-old child on Claritin? Are you happy running to the allergist twice a week to stick your 10-year-old with allergy injections? Are you scared that your child will have a fatal asthma attack on the playground? Perhaps your child is not even allowed on the playground because of their condition. Do you worry every time you or your child get sick that you will have to go on steroids or breathing treatments? This is a big deal, whether it is annoying itching, chronic sneezing, or bronchial passages closing. These symptoms are indications of much deeper issues, and if not corrected, things likely will become worse. Allergies and all that goes along with them can be reversed. After all, have you ever heard of a lion with an allergy? Do birds sneeze in the spring? Are some squirrels allergic to nuts?

News flash…Cheerios are not food! They are highly processed grains that must be pulverized, cooked, and flavored in order to be fit for consumption. Cow's milk is not food for a human (see the *duh* about protein), it is food for a calf. Artificial colors, flavors, and sweeteners are...artificial! Big duh there. Flesh of an animal is something we must kill, flavor, and cook to consume when there is nothing else to eat! Stop complicating your nutrition and your health issues; simplify, detoxify, and C.U.R.E.

Duh #12: "I don't have time to detox." You don't have time to NOT DETOX!!!

There is rarely a perfect time to get sick, have a baby, buy a new car, or change careers. There are occasions when some of these things are planned, but for many of us, they happen when they are going to happen and oftentimes we find ourselves just going with the flow!

Trust me, November 6, 2010 was not a good time to have a thyroid storm. Come to think of it, if given the opportunity, I likely would have never scheduled it. But, like Christmas (in the Dr. Seuss classic, *The Grinch Who Stole Christmas*), "it came just the same." As a practitioner of acupuncture and natural therapies, one would think that I would go out of my way to make time to clean up my body periodically. Nevertheless, I was usually too busy taking care of other people's bodies. Too busy to give mine a second glance (you know, cobbler's kid's shoes). As they say, hindsight is 20/20. As for now, I can tell you this, I will never give disease an opportunity to sneak up on me again, and neither should you!

There is ALWAYS time to detox. If you have time to eat, you have time to detox. Eating fruits and vegetables and taking some herbs takes up no more time than making a pot of coffee or running through the drive through of your local heart attack joint. Time is not the factor here. Love of yourself and commitment to your health is the main factor. If your husband, mother, or child suddenly became ill with a very serious disease, I guarantee you would make the time to care for them. You would rearrange your work schedule, find a carpool, or send all of your laundry to the local cleaners so that you can take your mom for surgery or your child for therapy. You would do what it takes for those you love, but what about yourself? Do you love yourself? Are you not important? Aren't you sick of feeling tired, moody, pain-filled, foggy-headed, and overweight? Do you resent being the science experiment of the next doctor you see? Don't you want to have control? Don't you want to feel empowered?

If the answer to any these questions is yes, then make the time to do something about it! Say it with me! DUH!!!

Tonight, take a look at your schedule and make time to go to the local grocery store or farmer's market and gather up a basket of life!

Duh #13: "I don't believe in alternative medicine."

Neither do I! Seriously, I totally do not believe in alternative medicine. But first let me define the word "alternative."

Let's say you're diagnosed with a disease. God forbid, but pretend it is cancer. You go to the Mayo clinic and their premier oncologist meets with you to discuss your treatment. The process involves having a major body part surgically removed after which you will undergo a therapy that includes slowly dripping a combination of acid chemicals into your veins that will cause severe flu-like symptoms with fever and chills, vomiting, headaches, and extreme fatigue. These symptoms will be addressed with other acidic medications. Your red and white blood cell count will plummet, causing you to require more drugs and possibly a blood transfusion. You will lose all of your hair and most likely a great deal of weight. You will appear as if you aged 10 years and you will feel as if it were 20. Your appetite will disappear, which will be addressed with more drugs and a strong recommendation for you to eat anything you like in order to put on weight, including ice cream, burgers, and French fries. You will be advised against eating raw fruits or vegetables as they may contain (normal) bacteria which your body may not be able to fight due to the devastation of your immune system by the drugs used to "heal" you and "kill" the cancer. When this treatment plan proves futile, the big guns of radiation are brought in to "burn" the cancer away. Hold on, weren't we taught to stay away from radiation? Doesn't radiation *cause* cancer? The process that I just described is how I define "alternative" medicine and should be held as the LAST alternative in the treatment of disease. It should not be used as the primary therapy. It should only be considered when all else fails!

As far as primary therapy goes for nearly all diseases including cancer (detailed in Chapter 8), here are the basic steps to take:

1. Eliminate all chemicals from the home, including household cleaning products, laundry detergents and room deodorizers, as well as all chemical body care products such as toothpaste, deodorant, mouthwash, shampoo, moisturizers etc. and replace them with all natural products. Simple things like baking soda and coconut oil can replace many body care products while vinegar, baking soda, and aroma therapy oils can replace household cleaning products. When it is time to paint the interior or exterior walls of your home, choose an eco-friendly paint. My favorite is Mythic paint (see resources).

2. Alkalize the diet 100% and detoxify the body with herbs.

3. Rediscover nature. Go the beach, the park, the mountains, and the forest and breathe in life force.

4. Pray, meditate, practice yoga, and incorporate stress-relieving habits into your lifestyle.

5. Exercise.

6. Love everything!

7. Repeat.

Understand that cutting, poisoning, and burning the body to address disease is the definition of insanity. Remember? Doing what you always did and expecting a different result. Modern cancer therapy is a bigger and more excessive example of the acid life you are already living. This should not be primary therapy.

So by my definition of alternative medicine, I agree, I do not believe in it. *Duh!*

"When the student is ready the teacher will appear.
When the student is truly ready...
The teacher will Disappear."

- Lao Tzu

C | U | R | E *quotes*

chapter eight
Steps to C.U.R.E.

The process of Cultivating Unlimited Rejuvenating Energy involves a deep detoxification and cellular rejuvenation protocol. This not a trivial process, yet it is by no means an insurmountable task. But when I am asked if one can detoxify and rejuvenate their body of a pain, an ailment, or disease in one week, 21 days, or even one month my response is "How long do you think it took you to get sick?" As attached as we have become to the western medical mindset of feeling better quickly, if you are reading this book, I assume you understand to a large extent that feeling better by medicating and suppressing symptoms is *not* C.U.R.E.

All that you have read up until this point has likely brought you to the understanding that the path to illness was a long and arduous process. For most of us, it is probable that we have spent 10+ years cultivating a state of inflammation in our body which ultimately led to our diagnosis. Oftentimes, we feel that the moment of the diagnosis is the moment the disease began. After all, just last year your blood tests were perfect, mammogram was negative and urine analysis was normal. Yet a blood test just one year later reveals a different story. How can we wrap our head around such a seemingly sudden change? Think of it like this. If you planted an acorn 6 inches under the ground and it took 4 weeks before you saw a tiny sprout pushing its way through the soil, would you think that the tree just began life? Of course you wouldn't. During the previous 4 weeks, the shell of the acorn began to soften as the dampness in the earth released enzyme inhibitors. Shortly after that, the acorn split open as a tiny, almost hair-like green sprout began to work its way out of the seed. It continued to develop, pushing through the earth until that moment when it became visible to the world. Certainly that moment of recognition (diagnosis) was not the moment the plant began to grow (process of disease). Our continuous exposure to acids today leads us to the diagnosis of tomorrow.

In the modern world children (and yes, I detoxify children as well) are exposed to higher concentrations of acid-forming foods and toxic chemicals than ever before. This in turn leads to the inflammatory process starting much earlier and with greater intensity. When using iridology as a tool to examine genetic weaknesses, I am still astounded to view the structural differences of the eyes over only two generations.

Today, children are weaned on acid-forming non-foods. As a matter of fact, an extraordinary number of children are put on an acid diet long before weaning, when life-giving breast milk is substituted with highly processed commercial formulas. If a newborn baby today is lucky enough to get breast milk for at least six months of their life, some of the benefits of that breast milk are often thwarted by the introduction of finger foods like Goldfish crackers, cookies, teething biscuits, or mac-n-cheese. The rapid integration of these non-foods bring children to a state of acid-hell far more rapidly than we have seen in the history of mankind. The mere fact that children are being diagnosed with adult diseases like type II diabetes, autoimmune issues, or breast cancer (I actually heard on the news, just today, that an eight year old girl was diagnosed with aggressive breast cancer) screams to us that an acid lifestyle is unsustainable.

As we walk through this process together you may initially feel overwhelmed by the challenge. Despite this, taking it step by step and allowing yourself to embrace the process will bring you to the realization of how incredibly simple this detoxification truly is. Coupled with simplicity is the understanding of how exceedingly important it is to dig deep and stay the course. The length of time that one stays on the process of detoxification naturally varies, and working with a certified practitioner (see Chapter 14: "Resources") is the best way to know when to dig in and when to back off. This book is intended to give you the most accurate and detailed understanding of detoxification and rejuvenation.

STEP 1: Evaluate your health status

There are many ways to evaluate and assess the status of your health in order to decide if it is time for you to detoxify and rejuvenate your body. Of course, if you have a diagnosis from a medical doctor, chiropractor, naturopath, or acupuncture physician, you will have starting point. Yet, outside of a traditional medical diagnosis, there are other ways to determine the state of one's health and ascertain whether they should delve into detoxification. In my office, we use many tools to make this assessment, including previous medical diagnoses. While we also utilize other western forms of analysis such as blood tests, X-rays, and CAT scans, there are various natural methods of evaluation within the realm of traditional Chinese medicine. These can include tongue and pulse diagnoses, naturopathic iridology, not to mention a good, old fashioned lengthy conversation. However, I have found that one of the most profound methods of evaluating an individual's health status is the self-assessment survey (see Chapter 15: "Self-Assessment Survey"). This is the same survey that I filled out many years ago, for my first meeting with Dr. Morse, and it continues to be what I use in my office to this day.

This health survey is poised to be an eye opening experience for everyone who fills it out, but especially for those who do not think they are in need of detoxification. As you answer the questions you will begin to understand that the human body is not a straight line with various disconnected body parts, but a sophisticated and intricate spider web, where one area of weakness leads to another and the source of one health issue in the body can be a direct result of the malfunction of another. For instance, having varicose or spider veins may be regarded as unsightly, but not a health issue to be concerned with from the viewpoint of western medicine. On the other hand, as you fill out the self-assessment survey, you will find that spider veins may be directly related to a weakness of the parathyroid gland which is in charge of regulating the usage of calcium in the body. Calcium is a very important component of blood vessel walls, supporting their integrity. A weakness in the function of the parathyroid could in fact be a cause of these vein issues. (There are other mechanisms as well such as malabsorption, over acidity, or deficient nutritional intake, but no matter what the foundational cause(s), the survey begins to put the pieces of the puzzle together so that the cause of the issue can finally be addressed.)

As these pieces of the evaluation process fall together, we will map out a plan of action. The plan will determine which issues should be the primary focus of the detoxification and which will be auxiliary. It will always include nutritional changes and an herbal protocol. We will also make decisions as to whether homeopathic remedies or animal glandular supplements are appropriate. Finally, the assessment will help us to determine if supportive therapies such as acupuncture, chiropractic, cranial sacral therapy, or lymphatic drainage are applicable. These therapies will be discussed in greater detail in Chapter 9: "Supportive treatment modalities."

STEP 2: Making dietary changes

Once the assessment is completed and a plan is created we can begin to initiate the detoxification protocol. Here is where we get into the meat and potatoes (pun totally intended) of detoxification. As stated in previous chapters, it is virtually impossible to reverse disease without completely going to the alkaline side of chemistry. However, for those of you who seek to challenge this topic with stories of how a friend lowered their blood pressure, reduced their cholesterol, or minimized joint pain on the South Beach, Blood-Type, or Paleo diets, I am not here to argue their success. You see, in today's extremely sick society, with lifestyles laden with processed food and food-like products it is not a surprise that if you follow any one of these diets, you can improve your numbers and even feel better. Why, you ask? Because every one of these diets removes some of the most destructive acid forming foods on the planet. They all tend to remove processed food, fried food, hydrogenated oils, chemical colors, preservatives, processed sugar, and sugar substitutes. The body becomes so unburdened by removing these acid toxins that it responds with great enthusiasm. And in some cases, especially where there is a very strong genetic lineage as determined through iridology photos, that may be all it takes to achieve a certain level of reversal.

But, as you learned in Chapter 2: "The Science of Sickness," while symptoms are the *first* things to go, their disappearing act is not a determining factor in the reversal of disease. High blood pressure is just a symptom. High cholesterol is just a symptom. And again, joint pain is just a symptom. There are many drugs on the market today that can alleviate these symptoms (what I call "symptoms" are referred to in western medicine as diseases), however the absence of symptoms is NOT an indication of the absence of disease. Yes, it may feel wonderful to minimize or erase a symptom with a drug. Does that mean the *cause* of the symptom is gone? The cause of illness is no more gone after taking a drug than it is by removing some acid from the diet. The cause of disease can only be reversed when you strip the body of long-term acid waste within the lymphatic system and support the organs of elimination and the glands of the endocrine system. This is accomplished via detoxification by completely removing all acid forming foods from the diet and establishing an appropriate herbal protocol.

The dietary changes during detoxification (we will discuss just how long the detoxification process will last later in this chapter) can be radical for some and nominal for others. No matter how you look at it, the importance of being determined and meticulous regarding your diet is enormous. If you are anything like me, you want your health crisis to be over yesterday! That being said, dabbling in detox is useless. You are either all in or not in at all.

Let's begin. In this detoxification diet we are going to remove particular foods for two reasons.

1. The food is acid-forming which ultimately congests the lymphatic system, leading to inflammation and disease as we discussed in previous chapters.

2. High protein sources, even when plant-based, will further bog down kidney function. Keep in mind that the kidneys play a huge part of the filtration and elimination of cellular waste and protein metabolism. Therefore, while on detox, one of the goals is to lighten the load of waste as much as possible in an effort to give the kidneys a break. Protein places a heavy load on the kidneys. Consequently, by removing high protein foods from the diet, the kidneys can

keep most of their focus on filtering waste that has been stagnant in the lymphatic system for years.

Now that the reasoning behind removing certain foods during a detoxification diet is clear, here is a list of food and food products that will be eliminated.

- All animal protein. This includes beef, pork, poultry, wild game, and eggs.

- All dairy and products made from dairy such as kefir, cheese, ice cream, and yogurt.

- All grains and grain products including rice (brown or white), quinoa, amaranth, bulgur, barley, corn etc. as well as all products made with grain, e.g. bread, pasta, baked goods, crackers etc.

- All nuts and seeds as well as nut butters and spreads.

- All beans except green beans.

- All processed and bottled oils including olive oil, almond oil, coconut oil etc.

- All types of salt including sea and Himalayan, as well bottled dressings, sauces, and condiments that contain salt.

- Black, white, and hot peppers.

- Cranberries and blueberries.

What to include in a detoxification diet:
- All fruits including but not limited to dried, fresh, or frozen fruit:

  o Sweet fruits: Bananas, dates, figs, grapes, jackfruit, jujube, longan, mamey sapote, mangosteen, papaya, persimmon

  o Sub-acid fruits: Apples, blackberries, cherimoya, cherries, grapes (seeded), loquat, lychee, mango, nectarine, peach, pear, plum, raspberries, blackberries

- o Acid-fruits: Cranberry, grapefruit, kiwi, kumquat, lemon, limes, oranges, pineapple, pomegranate, strawberry, tangerine, tomato (heirlooms are best)

- o Melons: Cantaloupe, watermelon, honeydew, and papayas can be in this category as well, as they are known as tree-melons.

- o Non-sweet fruits: Bell peppers and cucumber

- o High fat fruits: Avocado, durian, and olives (unsalted)

- o Starchy fruits: Zucchini, butternut squash, acorn squash, spaghetti squash etc.

- o Any other fruit not mentioned above.

- All vegetables including those that are found in the above "fruit" categories such as squash and the only bean allowed on detox—the green bean.

- Raw food as much as possible up to 100% (see menus below)

- Limited amount of cooked vegetables

- No cooked tomatoes

- Nightshades can be avoided if there is a known issue with them. Nightshades include eggplant, peppers, tomatoes, non-sweet potatoes, and goji berries

To those who live on a limited diet of animal protein (in the form of flesh, eggs, or dairy) and processed starches, the list of "allowed" foods may appear to be quite short. But, upon closer examination, you will find that the totality of these two food groups (fruit and vegetables) is so large that if you wanted to try one of every edible plant out there every week, you would likely not have enough time in your life. For example, there are over 100 types of mangoes, 1,600 types of bananas and 7,500 types of apples in the world! And while the place where you reside does not grow or import the vast majority of them, there is enough variety in your area to keep you detoxing, healthy, and interested in your meal, once you are exposed to them and the thousands of ways to combine and prepare them.

Speaking of food preparation, please note that Chapter 14: "Recipes and resources" will provide you with plenty of recipes to get you started, as well as direct you to valuable websites for great meal ideas. As long as you follow the parameters mentioned above, you can scan any vegan recipe online and make it detox friendly.

A little bit about food-combining
Many practitioners of natural therapies and nutritional healing often talk about the benefits of proper food combining. In my own practice, I have seen patients exhibit profoundly positive effects, including losing quite a few pounds, just by re-combining their foods according to some basic principles. Certainly there are those on the opposite side of this concept who believe that food combinations do not matter since it "all ends up in the same place anyway." I beg to differ and here is why.

The human body has one stomach which is divided into three sections. They are the fundus, the body, and the pylorus. Once you bite into a raw food such as an apple, the process of digestion begins. In the mouth, mechanical digestion known as chewing or mastication is initiated which is immediately followed by the secretion of the digestive enzyme, amylase, by the salivary glands. On some occasions the salivary glands secrete amylase *before* one even takes a bite of food. For example, the act of cutting a lemon will cause a simultaneous release of saliva or "mouth-watering." Once food is placed in the mouth and mastication begins, amylase gets mixed in with the morsel of food and aids in its breakdown.

As food is swallowed, entering the esophagus and then the stomach, the body is alerted that certain enzymes, gastric juices, and stomach acid are needed to further break down the food. Different amounts of stomach acid and various enzymes ratios are required for each type of food. When food consumption is kept simple, digestion is timely and effortless. But when many different types of food are combined in one meal or consumed too close together, the digestion process can become overburdened and arduous. Let me give you an example.

There is no doubt that wrapping a piece of prosciutto around a slice of cantaloupe will not kill you (well not immediately anyway!). But the combination of these two foods are likely to cause an eruption of fumes from one or two ends of your body that could bring Arnold Schwarzenegger to his knees. Flatulence, or "gas" as most of us call it, is a reaction inside the body that is *common* but not *normal*. At least it is not normal in the amounts in which humans tend to produce it, requiring over-the-counter medications like Gas-X or Pepto Bismol. I am quite sure that there is someone that will argue this point, but as they say, the proof is in the pudding.

Since different foods break down at various rates with different levels of enzymes and stomach acid, food that takes the shortest time to process (cantaloupe) will sit in the stomach while food that takes longer (prosciutto) continues to be processed. Let's get a visual.

Imagine if you will, both the cantaloupe and prosciutto sitting on a hot asphalt road in the middle of July in Phoenix, Arizona. As each hour passes, a photo is taken of the food lying on the street. From one photo to the next, over the course of 10 hours, the degradation of the two pieces of food becomes obvious. By the next afternoon, the cantaloupe is a goopy, broken down heap, impossible to pick up with your fingers. On the other hand, the prosciutto, though inedible, still maintains its integrity. This is what happens in your 98.6 °F stomach. While the animal flesh is still in need of the digestive process, the fruit is finished. But, since they were eaten together, the fruit must remain in the stomach until the breakdown of the animal product is complete. The fruit begins to ferment within the confines of the stomach and gas gets produced as a byproduct of fermentation and as you know, gas can wreak all kinds of havoc in the realm of belching, burping and yes, flatulence (scientifically known as farting). Besides the unseemly effects of improper food combining, there is also the issue of poor absorption of nutrition through the wall of the small intestine leading to nutritional deficiencies and deficient syndromes.

Practicing food combining for just seven days can greatly change the volume and potency of the gas that you produce, thereby allowing digestion and absorption to be more effective and efficient. Not to mention, keeping everyone around you happy too! You don't have to take my word for it. Just try it for a week or two and see what happens.

I have happened across those rare individuals (who are the exception, not the rule) whose gas production increases when they first embark on a fruit and vegetable diet. It may take two or three weeks to resolve by just sticking to the process or that person's digestive system may need a little support. If that is the case, the cause of excess gas production will be addressed with the appropriate herbs or glandular supplementation. These herbs or glandular pills will only be used until the issue is resolved. But make no mistake about it, flatulence of any magnitude should be resolved.

The actual practice of food combining is certainly used during detoxification and can easily be carried over into a maintenance plan once the detoxification phase is completed. This will allow for ease of digestion in several ways:
- The reduction or elimination of gas, bloating, and belching

- Elimination of acid reflux and heart burn

- Greater absorption of nutrition

- A feeling of satisfaction from food

- Elimination of cravings

It is always important to maintain optimal digestion both during and after detoxification. While there may be times that proper food combining becomes a challenge (for example in social situations such as eating in restaurants, holidays or events) the majority of the time it is quite easy to follow. Your digestive tract and your body will thank you for a job well done! I have included a post-detoxification food combining chart for once detox is complete.

Both the detoxification and post-detoxification food combining charts are designed to be easy to follow and while it would be impossible to list every food in each category box, you can clearly get a sense of the types of food that belongs within each category.

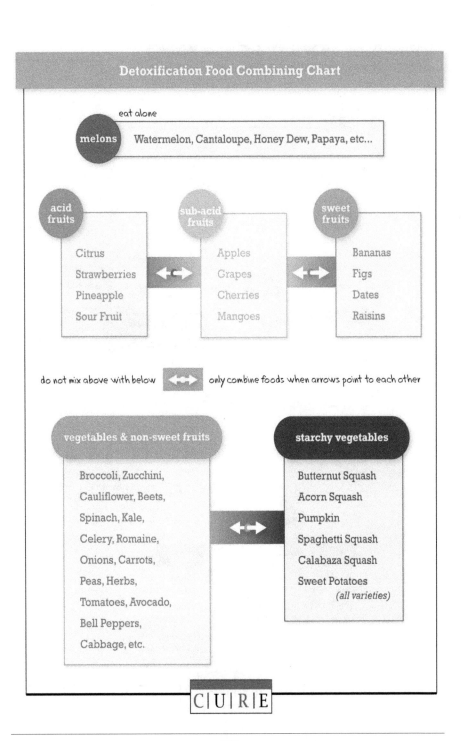

Detoxification Food Combining Chart

eat alone

melons — Watermelon, Cantaloupe, Honey Dew, Papaya, etc...

acid fruits

Citrus
Strawberries
Pineapple
Sour Fruit

sub-acid fruits

Apples
Grapes
Cherries
Mangoes

sweet fruits

Bananas
Figs
Dates
Raisins

do not mix above with below — only combine foods when arrows point to each other

vegetables & non-sweet fruits

Broccoli, Zucchini,
Cauliflower, Beets,
Spinach, Kale,
Celery, Romaine,
Onions, Carrots,
Peas, Herbs,
Tomatoes, Avocado,
Bell Peppers,
Cabbage, etc.

starchy vegetables

Butternut Squash
Acorn Squash
Pumpkin
Spaghetti Squash
Calabaza Squash
Sweet Potatoes
(all varieties)

C | U | R | E

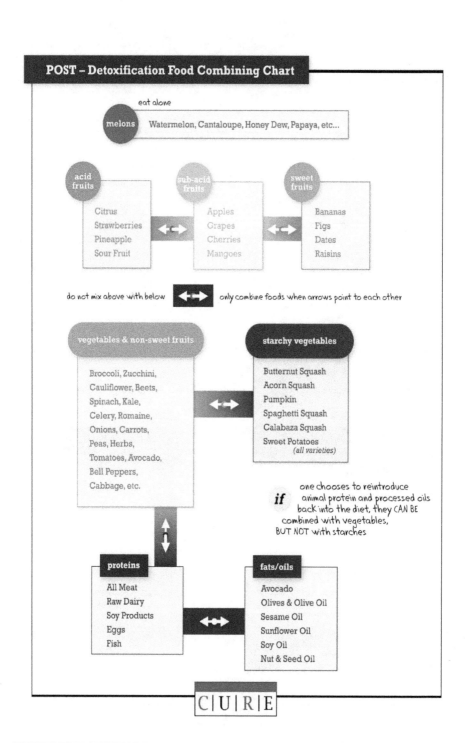

POST – Detoxification Food Combining Chart

melons — eat alone
Watermelon, Cantaloupe, Honey Dew, Papaya, etc...

acid fruits
Citrus
Strawberries
Pineapple
Sour Fruit

sub-acid fruits
Apples
Grapes
Cherries
Mangoes

sweet fruits
Bananas
Figs
Dates
Raisins

do not mix above with below   only combine foods when arrows point to each other

vegetables & non-sweet fruits
Broccoli, Zucchini,
Cauliflower, Beets,
Spinach, Kale,
Celery, Romaine,
Onions, Carrots,
Peas, Herbs,
Tomatoes, Avocado,
Bell Peppers,
Cabbage, etc.

starchy vegetables
Butternut Squash
Acorn Squash
Pumpkin
Spaghetti Squash
Calabaza Squash
Sweet Potatoes
(all varieties)

if one chooses to reintroduce animal protein and processed oils back into the diet, they CAN BE combined with vegetables, BUT NOT with starches

proteins
All Meat
Raw Dairy
Soy Products
Eggs
Fish

fats/oils
Avocado
Olives & Olive Oil
Sesame Oil
Sunflower Oil
Soy Oil
Nut & Seed Oil

C | U | R | E

Timing rule of thumb

After having a fruit meal it is a good idea to wait at least one hour before eating vegetables. After eating a vegetable meal it is best to wait two to four hours before eating fruits again. These are general guidelines, but the greatest judge is your own digestive system. If you experience gas, belching, bloating, or any digestive discomfort, be sure to wait longer before consuming a dissimilar food.

How much food should I eat and how often?

When one is "dieting" there is frequently a question about the necessary quantity of food and timing of meals. How much should I eat? What is a serving of vegetables, fruit, or protein? How often should I eat? Should I eat three large meals or six small ones? On and on it goes, trying to discover the magic formula to calories, carbs, fats, and proteins. We get so wrapped up in these uncertainties that we fail to notice our bodies. We rely on our wrist watch or a cell phone app to tell us when to eat, instead of asking our *cells!* You remember your cells. The 100 trillion little parts which you consist of, along with blood and lymph! They are the ones in charge. It is their needs that must be met, not your app, watch, or food journal's.

Getting in touch with your cells is key to transforming the way you look at food and ultimately, your health. But it does take a bit of time to really be able to tap into what your cells are telling you. This is especially true if you have been eating unconsciously for so many years, grabbing this or that, eating because others are eating, because it is "lunch time," or because you are feeling sad that day. Due to our history of eating habits I would like to offer a little direction. That is, until you develop the insight you need to listen to your body.

During the first week of detoxification, I highly recommend that you not allow yourself to get truly hungry. You know that feeling. When you walk in the door after a long day, you had toast and coffee for breakfast, half a bagel with some melted creamy stuff for lunch and a handful of trail mix with *real* M&M's for an afternoon snack. By the time you arrive home you are ravenous and even the dog treats look appealing. When detoxing, this is a huge no-no, especially during week one when you are trying to navigate through this new way of life while still living in your old one. Of course bagels, trail mix, and coffee are out, but given the amount of foods on the "yes" list how much should you eat? As much as you want and as much as it takes to keep you from feeling hungry. I want you to eat like a monkey!

I found that during my first week of detox, having a bowl of grapes, cut up watermelon, or carrots with guacamole helped me to stay on track and not get hungry. Between the chewing, incredible amount of hydration (often times thirst is mistaken for hunger), massive amount of nutrition, and natural sugar for cellular energy, you may arrive home from your busy day barely interested in dinner. My advice, wait a little while and then have dinner. I'd rather you feel a bit full that first week, than have you wake up at 1:00 a.m. looking for a snack.

By week two you can slow down a bit, and by week three you will be amazed by how small amounts of food can satisfy you. The menus below are a guideline. There will be days when you wish to eat more frequently and days when you only want fruit smoothies. Pay attention, listen, and trust. Do not, however trust the little voice inside that is whispering *"pizza."* That is your old self that pops up now and then. Make a smoothie or spaghetti squash with sun-dried tomatoes, basil, and oregano and press on!

Next you will find three menus labeled *Phase 1, Phase 2 and Phase 3*. They represent 3 levels of detoxification. If you consume the standard American diet, I recommend that you follow phase 1 for at least 1–2 weeks before moving to phase 2 and then 3. Each phase takes you to a deeper level of detoxification. Along with each level may be an increased amount or intensity of detoxification symptoms (these will be discussed later in this chapter). At any time during detox, you can "lighten up" the detox symptoms by backing off a phase. That means if you are on phase 3 and you experience headaches that make it difficult for you to work, you can go down to phase 1. By adding in some vegetables, your detox symptoms can ease a bit. Keep in mind that all detox symptoms are temporary and will abate. Therefore, lightening up on the menu is not mandatory, but a personal choice. Learn to listen to your body and make wise decisions.

breakfast

You may choose from any group and eat whole or blend in a smoothie. There is no restriction of quantity.

berries
Blackberries
Blueberries
Raspberries
Strawberries

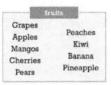

fruits	
Grapes	
Apples	Peaches
Mangos	Kiwi
Cherries	Banana
Pears	Pineapple

melons
Watermelon
Papaya
Cantaloupe
Honey Dew
Canary Melon

mid-morning snack

Fruit, fresh fruit juice, fresh green juice.

lunch

Create a wonderful salad with these or any other raw, unprocessed vegetables.

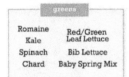

greens	
Romaine	Red/Green
Kale	Leaf Lettuce
Spinach	Bib Lettuce
Chard	Baby Spring Mix

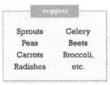

veggies	
Sprouts	Celery
Peas	Beets
Carrots	Broccoli,
Radishes	etc.

non-sweet fruits
Cucumber
Avocado
Bell Peppers
Zucchini

mid-afternoon snack

If you choose fruit, please allow at least 2 hours for proper digestion of lunch.

Fruit, fresh fruit juice, fresh green juice.

dinner

Large Salad
PLUS a small serving of either:

Steamed Vegetables Veggie Soup, or Baked Sweet Potato, or Steamed Squash, OR Avocado

• Please keep in mind that starchy vegetables such as squash and sweet potatoes are mucus forming and should be kept to a minimum.

Please see our RECIPES for entrees or dressing suggestions.

C | U | R | E

breakfast

You may choose chose from any group and eat whole or blend in a smoothie. There is no restriction of quantity.

berries
Blackberries
Blueberries
Raspberries
Strawberries

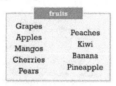

fruits	
Grapes	Peaches
Apples	Kiwi
Mangos	Banana
Cherries	Pineapple
Pears	

melons
Watermelon
Papaya
Cantaloupe
Honey Dew
Canary Melon

mid-morning snack   Fruit, fresh fruit juice, fresh green juice.

lunch

You may choose chose from any group and eat whole or blend in a smoothie. There is no restriction of quantity.

berries
Blackberries
Blueberries
Raspberries
Strawberries

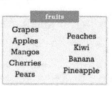

fruits	
Grapes	Peaches
Apples	Kiwi
Mangos	Banana
Cherries	Pineapple
Pears	

melons
Watermelon
Papaya
Cantaloupe
Honey Dew
Canary Melon

mid-afternoon snack

If you choose fruit, please allow at least 2 hours for proper digestion of lunch.

Fruit, fresh fruit juice, fresh green juice.

dinner

Large Salad
PLUS a small serving of either:

Steamed Vegetables, Steamed Squash, OR Avocado

Please see our RECIPES for entrees or dressing suggestions.

C|U|R|E

breakfast

You may choose chose from any group and eat whole or blend in a smoothie. There is no restriction of quantity.

berries
Blackberries
Blueberries
Raspberries
Strawberries

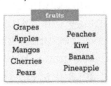

fruits	
Grapes	
Apples	Peaches
Mangos	Kiwi
Cherries	Banana
Pears	Pineapple

melons
Watermelon
Papaya
Cantaloupe
Honey Dew
Canary Melon

mid-morning snack   Fruit, fresh fruit juice, fresh green juice.

lunch

You may choose chose from any group and eat whole or blend in a smoothie. There is no restriction of quantity.

berries
Blackberries
Blueberries
Raspberries
Strawberries

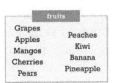

fruits	
Grapes	
Apples	Peaches
Mangos	Kiwi
Cherries	Banana
Pears	Pineapple

melons
Watermelon
Papaya
Cantaloupe
Honey Dew
Canary Melon

mid-afternoon snack

If you choose fruit, please allow at least 2 hours for proper digestion of lunch.

Fruit, fresh fruit juice, fresh green juice.

dinner   You may choose chose from any group and eat whole or blend in a smoothie. There is no restriction of quantity.

berries
Blackberries
Blueberries
Raspberries
Strawberries

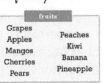

fruits	
Grapes	
Apples	Peaches
Mangos	Kiwi
Cherries	Banana
Pears	Pineapple

melons
Watermelon
Papaya
Cantaloupe
Honey Dew
Canary Melon

• Large Salad (optional) & no more than 3x/week.

A note about water

Following the line of questioning *"how much?"* it is important to address the topic of water and hydration. The belief that there is a science to how much and how often we should eat has led us to the concept that the amount of water we drink should be determined by a mathematical equation. There are actually web sites that ask questions varying from your height and weight, to how much you sweat to determine how many ounces of water you should drink per hour. How fragile we have become with this need to walk around with our water bottles just to make it to our next destination? Does all of this make sense or does it seem that someone is gaining from our necessity to be hydrated? This could have been a question for the *Duh* chapter, but I think we can address it here.

There is no doubt in my mind that modern humans are regularly in a dehydrated state. The question is why? Why are we thirsty? Why do we own a collection of BVT free water bottles? When did cars start having cup holders and humans start hauling liquid? The answer lies in chemistry. Yes, it goes back to that acid/alkaline balance. The more acidic we are, the more we burn up fluids and tissues in our body. In an acidic state, the body needs more and more water to buffer its effects and in essence put out the fire. On a natural diet (detox and post-detox), the body no longer requires water as you know it. Not in the form of cups, bottles, and glasses. The cleanest, most alkaline, and greatest source of water the human body could obtain comes directly from...your diet! Fruit and vegetables contain practically all of the water your body needs, wants, or could use. As long as you satisfy your caloric needs with these foods in their raw state, you should not need to lug around that bottle of water. Keep in mind there are certainly exceptions to this concept. For example, the more cooked food, spicy food, salty food, or condensed food (white potatoes vs. peaches) you consume the more hydration you will need. We tend to drink either during or after a meal that is salty, spicy, or cooked. Also keep in mind that exercise and physical activity will increase your need for hydration. I tend to eat fruit before yoga class or a long trek with my dog. Yet, I must be sure to time my intake of food wisely as performing a headstand in yoga does not bode well with a full belly. If water becomes a better choice due to activity, transport, or availability, by all means I will drink water. However, as you delve deeper into detoxification you will be amazed at how little you actually "drink." This is a learning process and a practice of discovery. Whether you are eating for calories or hydration, it is important that you learn to feel the effects of food on your cells and allow that feeling to drive your decision to eat or drink.

Physical manifestations of detoxification

Of course, our goal in terms of physical manifestations of detoxification is to reverse the causes of disease and C.U.R.E. within the body, thus eliminating those physical issues. Unfortunately, detoxification is not a linear process taking us easily from point A to point B. Detoxification is a meandering, winding road with ups and downs and sometimes fender-benders!

In the midst of the detoxification process, all sorts of feelings can arise. They range from physical sensations to emotional changes and anything in between. Now don't go getting scared. No one has died from detox! But it is important to understand just what is going on in the body and what you can do to ease the possible manifestations of detoxification.

First off, let's talk about what is going on in the body when someone embarks on detoxification. In the last year or so, science has discovered the glymphatic system. This is the lymphatic system of the brain. (You remember the lymphatic system we discussed oh so many chapters ago?). The glymphatic system does for the brain what the lymphatic system does for the rest of the body. It is the sewer system, collecting cellular waste to be transported to the lymph nodes and then processed for removal via the kidneys, colon and skin.

In the discovery of the glymphatic system, scientists revealed that the brain primarily detoxifies itself at night when we sleep (Iliff et al., 2012)! This uncovered enormously important information regarding insomnia, sleep deprivation, and the connection to several diseases including high blood pressure, diabetes, and dementia. Neuroscientists at the University of Rochester Medical Center (Xie, 2013) have also found that during nighttime sleep brain cells actually contract, squeezing out metabolic waste, much like squeezing dirty water from a sponge. This toxic waste from cells will cause damage if left in or around them (inflammation→degeneration→disease). As discovered by traditional Chinese medicine thousands of years ago, different tissues of the body optimize function, clean themselves, rest, and eliminate waste at different times of the day. This is known as the circadian clock. It is a magnificent system, and when the body is in an alkaline state, the process of removing toxins from the cells is relatively unnoticed and uneventful. However, when the body has been in an acidic state for months, years, or decades, the ability to eliminate these toxins is significantly reduced, until…the implementation of detoxification! Once a 100% alkaline diet and vital herbs are introduced, the cellular detoxification process gets kicked into overdrive!

What does that mean for you? Old injury sites of hardened scar tissue and unnecessary cells begin to break down, only to rebuild and regenerate new and more viable ones. This can cause discomfort and even cycles of pain. When I was detoxifying, I developed pain on my left sacrum and right pubic bone. As I struggled to figure out what I had done that day to cause my pains, I remembered the conversation I had with Dr. Morse during our first meeting. He showed me how my eyes (via iridology which will be covered later in this chapter) revealed prior injuries to my pelvis! He was right on the mark! Just a few years prior to getting diagnosed with Graves' disease I had fallen (actually flown) off of my horse and hit a steel pole before crashing to the ground. The end result? A double pelvic fracture involving my left sacrum and right anterior pelvic bones causing me to be wheelchair-bound for nearly five weeks. The old injury that I had long forgotten reared its ugly head. This is better known as a healing crisis which eventually leads to cellular restructuring. The pain, which was more appropriately described as intermittent discomfort, only lasted a week or so, just in time to move on to something new. This is why I love using iridology with my patients. It serves as a window into the future, allowing me the ability to "predict" what parts of the body will feel pain or show symptoms during the detoxification and rejuvenation process!

Again, to ease your mind, detox symptoms or healing crises are by no means continuous and ongoing. They ebb and flow like ocean tides, with many days bringing absolutely calm seas. There is no guarantee that you will experience discomfort. Though that may cause you to breathe a sigh of relief, I have actually had patients complain intensely within the first 2–3 weeks of detoxification that they still had not experienced a healing crisis! Wow, now I even have complaints for feeling good!

Aside from stirring up old injuries, a healing crisis could resemble other health issues you may have had in the past or even exacerbate the current issues that you are detoxing for. For example, maybe you had allergies as a child, but with numerous suppressant medications, your symptoms have gone away. You stopped experiencing headaches, a runny nose, or itchy eyes. Yet, two weeks into a clean diet and herbal formulas, your old allergy symptoms begin to awaken. Your nose begins to run after taking the herbs or maybe when you eat. You start sneezing or develop a little cough and wonder if you are allergic to the herbs? You contemplate the possibility that a detox diet isn't good for you. After all, you don't have the blood type for a vegan diet! WRONG! You are not having these symptoms because you are allergic to herbs, can't eat fruits, or have a particular blood type. You are having these reactions because your body is very deeply cleaning house. Mark my words, these things are expected AND celebrated! In my office, we love to hear stories of skin rashes, mucus pouring from the nose, or sputum expectorated from the lungs. We love stories about funky sensations or weird things in the toilet (I will do my best to avoid details in this matter). There are literally dozens of stories I could share about healing crises, from headaches to fevers. These healing crises are not dangerous but they can sometimes feel uncomfortable.

In the next section you will see a list of commonly experienced healing crises and suggestions of how to deal with them. But before we move on to that list, I would like to discuss the emotional side of a healing crisis. There is no doubt that being sick with a chronic condition is no picnic. My run-in with Graves' disease was undoubtedly the worst physical experience of my life. I often said that I would trade one thyroid storm for ten pelvic fractures any day.

Emotions run high and wild during illness. Therefore it is important to understand that during detoxification, (especially if you are doing it because you are dealing with a serious illness), there are going to be emotional upheavals. These upheavals are not only related to cellular changes during detoxification but the release of cellular memories from long ago. This cellular overhaul is not limited to liver, kidney, or heart cells. ALL cells are involved in this process. The cells that play the greatest role in our emotions are connected to one of the most important systems of the human body on which we focus many of our detox herbs. That system is called the endocrine system.

A thorough description of the endocrine system is beyond the scope of this book. Instead we will examine the "Reader's Digest" version of this vital system. The endocrine system is the collection of glands that produce hormones which are secreted into the circulatory system, regulating actions such as metabolism, growth and development, tissue function, sexual function, reproduction, sleep, and mood, among other things. While the majority of the endocrine system regulates function, a portion of its actions directly effects our emotions.

Emotions such as irritability, depression, and anxiety all have roots in surges and imbalances of hormones. Thus, when undertaking detoxification, there are the somewhat anticipated physical symptoms like headaches or a runny nose, and then there are the unexpected emotional symptoms like weepiness or a short temper. But emotions are intertwined in cellular function and the cleansing process of one will likely uncover another. Once again, this is not a reason to avoid detoxification. Quite the contrary, it is a reason to delve deep into detoxification and rejuvenation and see how much brighter things are on the other side.

Here's one last note about emotional releases during detoxification. In a detox diet, you are consuming foods (especially in their raw state) that are of the highest vibration there is in the form of food. Food such as fresh fruit, especially if picked in your region and at the perfect state of ripeness, are filled with life and God-force. I am not one to get into preaching about spirituality (my preaching about detox keeps me busy enough), but I can say this with certainty. God, Elah, Elohim, Allah or nature, universal energy, or whatever name you choose, has given us the gift of all of the fruit that trees will bear. Fruits typically grow high in the branches of a tree or cover the outer branches of a bush and grow in the glory of sunlight. They are of the highest energetic vibration that we can put into our bodies, healing wounds, tearing apart tumors, and energizing the brain and nervous system. This energy touches our emotions on every level, from hormonal to vibrational and will change how you feel about…EVERYTHING! Understanding that emotional changes and releases are a welcome part of detoxification and looking forward to the rejuvenation of cells and balancing of emotions is just as important as healing a disease.

Healing crisis: Symptoms and what to do.

Digestive changes

What it feels like.
Digestive changes can include diarrhea, constipation, gas, bloating, and/or belching.

What it means.
These symptoms can mean several things. Always keep in mind that past symptoms may come up during detox or current symptoms may get worse. If these are the symptoms that you were having prior to starting detox, then you are in a healing crisis. These symptoms may also be a response to the high amount of plant fiber introduced into your body by the detox diet. This is a tremendous change from the S.A.D. (Standard American Diet) and once the movement ability of fiber comes in, there will likely be an opening of the flood gates. On the flip side, sometimes the addition of high amounts of alkaline food can temporarily have an opposite effect. The purging of acids from the lymphatic system can cause a backup effect, much like yelling "fire" in a movie theater. Everyone gets up at once and rushes the door causing gridlock. I'll address how to handle this below. Gas, bloating, and belching can be related to the significant increase of fibrous foods in the diet, as

well as improper food combining.

Should I stop detox?

Detox can be slowed or stopped if you feel extremely uncomfortable, become dehydrated, light-headed, or feel faint. While those issues are rare, you must use your discretion and common sense when deciding whether to continue or slow detoxification. The necessity to stop detoxification is rare and usually more of an emotional choice than a physical need. Note that digestive changes are the most common occurrence in detoxification.

What to do.

In the case of diarrhea, you can add in a baked sweet potato or red skin potato which will help bind things up. The appropriate herbs will also help ease any inflammation that may be part of the reason the body is purging. Increasing vegetables and decreasing fruits, thus slowing down the detox process will also quell diarrhea. If diarrhea has led to dehydration, you can slow the process by eating more cooked food or a little bit of brown rice. Blueberry tea or a mixture of carob powder in water will also help to ease diarrhea. Of course, be sure to hydrate with fresh fruit, a fruit smoothie, or coconut water. Do not use sports drinks. Once diarrhea is under control, begin to reduce the consumption of cooked vegetables and brown rice and increase raw food. It may take several days before you can be on a complete detox diet again.

Constipation can be alleviated by the proper herbs or the addition of more fruit.

Gas, bloating, and belching is often caused by improper food combining. Please refer to the Detox and Post Detox Food Combining Charts in this chapter and follow either one precisely. You may even introduce mono-meals for a period of time to give the digestive system a break. Mono meals are meals which consist of a single food. For example, breakfast might be only grapes while lunch may be only salad greens.

Cold and flu-like symptoms:

What it feels like.
Sneezing, runny nose, congestion, passing of a great deal of mucus from the sinus and nasal cavities, coughing, mild fever, sweats, chills, and/or body aches.

What it means.
Cold and flu-like symptoms are a sign of the body purging old waste. These symptoms are not necessarily from a cold and are looked upon as a rite of passage into detox. If you are exposed to someone with a viral infection, rejoice! A virus is an opportunity for the body to do a deep cleaning and eliminate stagnant acid waste. In modern society, these symptoms are frowned upon and much is done to subdue them with analgesics, medication to "dry up" congestion and mucus, or cough suppressants. But the body knows better, and the natural elimination of these symptoms with time serves the body well during the process of detoxification. A detox diet (with or without the aid of a virus) often causes these symptoms whose onset is important to the healing process.

Should I stop detox?
No, continue to allow the body to purge waste in this natural manner. If you feel extremely uncomfortable, detox can be slowed down by adding some cooked food, brown rice, or gluten-free crackers into the diet. Remember, this too shall pass and the more of the healing crisis you are able to "ride out," the better you will be in the long run. I am always cognizant of the fact that everyone has a different tipping point and you should honor yours. If a fever gets too

uncomfortable or goes on for too long, then an aspirin can be taken to ease the discomfort or to help you rest or sleep. This will not stop the process of detox nor reverse any of the progress you have made, but rather allow you to rest and fight another day.

What to do.

Rest. Use a neti pot or nasal flush (I like the NeilMed sinus rinse bottles) with tepid distilled water and a pinch of sea salt to rinse sinus and nasal cavities. Use aroma therapy oils like peppermint, eucalyptus, tea tree, or a commercial blend such as Doterra's Breath to comfortably open sinus and nasal cavities. Breathing essential oils through a diffuser, placing a few drops on a cotton ball or in a diluted mix with a carrier oil while making direct contact within or around the nasal passages are wonderful ways to use these oils. Please note the dilution ratio with a carrier oil like coconut or almond should be 20:1, i.e. 20 drops of coconut oil to one drop of peppermint.

Consume watermelon and grapes to ease fever and keep hydrated. If watermelon is not available, any melon will do. Citrus can also be effective. Seek medical attention if temperature exceeds 103 °F.

Body aches or pains.

What it feels like.

Body aches can coincide with cold and flu symptoms or can occur independently. These pains can vary in strength, intensity, duration, and type. Throbbing, aching, stabbing, sharp, or dull pains are all possible in muscles or joints.

What it means.

No matter what the pain type, they are all a result of purging waste from toxic tissues into the lymphatic system. Depending on your history, aches and pains may be a result of old injuries (e.g. severe sprains, strains, broken bones) or current issues including fibromyalgia, arthritis, or gout, just to name a few. Body pains during detox are very, very common and often celebrated as a great step in the right direction.

Should I stop detox?

No. Keep going! Again, this could be challenging, but know that it will ebb and flow and eventually pass.

What to do.

Warm baths in Epsom salts or essential oils (chamomile, lavender, eucalyptus, peppermint, sage juniper frankincense, or yarrow are all wonderful choices. Purchase them at your local health food store or on line, see Resources.) will go a long way to ease the discomfort of body pain.

Other wonderful ways to work through detox body pains or other detox symptoms are acupuncture, lymphatic drainage massage, cranial sacral therapy, sound therapy, and color therapy (see more about these in Chapter 9: "Supportive treatment modalities"), as well as specific herbal formulas for pain.

Vomiting

What it feels like.

Discomfort can range from feelings of nausea, to dry heaving, to actual vomiting. This is not common nor does it occur continuously if you do experience it. Some individuals may vomit due to herbal remedies or simply to the introduction of new foods. The vomiting of mucus is much more likely than that of ingested food. In the case of mucus, again this is toxic waste finding its way out of the body.

What it means.

If phlegm or mucus is being vomited, your body is expelling toxic waste. This is a positive response to detoxification.

If food is vomited more than once or twice, this may be a strong reaction to herbs if used and one must evaluate doses and when herbs are taken. Herb dose or frequency can be reduced and the consumption of food with herbs can be altered. This is best done with a practitioner.

Should I stop detox?
There is no need to stop the detox process if vomiting of mucus occurs. If foodstuffs are vomited more than twice, the strength and timing of herbs should be reevaluated by a natural practitioner. If you are working by yourself, and are taking herbs, be sure to reduce them to one dose per day. If vomiting persists, discontinue herbs for a week and then reintroduce them at a much lower dose. If you are not working with herbs, introduce some cooked food into the diet and slowly decrease cooked foods once vomiting has stopped.

What to do.
For nausea or vomiting, support the digestive system with fresh ginger root tea. Thinly slice a half inch piece of fresh ginger root. Add the ginger to two cups of boiling water and lower to a simmer for five minutes. Sip slowly and repeat as needed. Peppermint tea can be had as well.

Vomiting foodstuffs more than twice should result in:

- Reevaluating any herbal remedies and lowering amount of herbs taken in a dose. Take herbs after eating or with meals instead of before meals.

- Slow down juicing or blending and add in more steamed vegetables or sweet potato.

- Ward off dehydration by sipping on water with fresh squeezed lemon or orange juice.

- Seek medical attention if vomiting goes on for more than two days and the suggestions above have not alleviated these symptoms. It is not uncommon for the body to expel foodstuffs that are very different from your usual diet or for herbs to induce some amount of digestive discomfort. The digestive tract is more effected by prescription medications as well as herbal supplements than any other part of the body. Do not fear these natural responses by your body.

Fever

What it feels like.

Fever can be low grade, hot flashes, night sweats or a true high fever. It can result in a headache, body aches, or general feeling of malaise.

What it means.

The body causes fever for many reasons, including fighting germs, viruses, and bacteria. During detoxification the body may be fighting germs but fever is often a response to the purging of toxic substances. Again, this is a positive reaction by the body.

Should I stop detox?

Fever is not a reason to stop detox. It is uncomfortable, should be monitored and managed if necessary, but should be allowed to run its course for the most part. Detox will be stopped or slowed down only if the person becomes dehydrated, if the fever has gone on for more than three days, or if the fever rises above 103 °F.

What to do.

Rest, monitor temperature, stay well hydrated with fresh fruits, fruit juices, and lemon water. If fever persists, decrease herbs, eat cooked vegetables, soup, or brown rice. A cool bath or a cool cloth on the forehead, back of neck, abdomen, or inner legs and arms are very helpful. If fever persists for more than two days, take a light dose of aspirin (or another antipyretic that you are familiar with if there is an aspirin allergy) to lower the fever to a comfortable level until the fever has subsided.

Seek medical attention if the fever will not break after taking aspirin.

Medical attention can include an acupuncture physician, a medical doctor, urgent care, or emergency room.

Headaches

What it feels like.

Headaches may manifest as pressure, pounding, or throbbing. It may be one sided or encompass the entire head. Sinuses may be involved, or it may accompany cold-like symptoms. It may also be accompanied by the expectoration of mucus.

What it means.

The movement of stagnant lymphatic congestion through the head will cause any of the various types of headaches. Old injuries to the head, neck, or upper back may flare up during detox, leading to headache symptoms. Headaches can also be a result of low calorie intake (or low blood sugar) during detoxification due to dietary changes and not planning meals and snacks ahead of time.

The cessation of coffee, medications, alcohol, sugar,

salt, and/or smoking can also lead to headaches, especially in the first 1–2 weeks of detoxification.

Should I stop detox?

No, headaches are very common and should not be a reason to stop detoxification.

What to do.

Rest, drink plenty of fresh fruit or vegetable juice or water with lemon. Eat a great deal of fruits. Make sure that you are consuming enough calories.

Have a few acupuncture, lymphatic drainage, or cranial sacral treatments. A chiropractic adjustment may also be indicated.

Heartburn/reflux

What it feels like.

Burning, pressure, or pain in the area of the upper stomach or in the esophagus.

What it means.

Even though this is a 100% alkaline diet, there can be acid-like effects from eating so much produce, especially in the case of the S.A.D. (Standard American Diet). The body is so used to consuming processed foods with no fiber or nutritional value that it is shocked by fresh, whole, and live food. Certain fruits, while having an alkaline effect on the cells, can feel acidic in the stomach. Oranges, pineapple, and grapefruit may initially have this effect. This will eventually pass.

Another common culprit is improper food combining. Please see the food combining chart in the early part of this chapter.

Should I stop detox?

No. This is a common occurrence and is not a reason to stop detoxification.

What to do.

Pay very close attention to proper food combinations. Some individuals are more prone to issues with improper food combining than others. This may be a weak area that needs extra attention.

Avoid more acidic fruits (such as citrus or pineapple) for a period of time until digestion improves.

A tablespoon of apple cider vinegar or baking soda mixed with water once or twice a day may be helpful for a short period of time.

Low energy

What it feels like.

Low energy is a very subjective term. For some, it may have been an issue prior to detox which continues to persist. For others it may be a new occurrence which may ebb and flow throughout the detox process. It is characterized as sleepiness, a heaviness in the limbs, or a foggy mind. It may also feel like a lack of motivation.

What it means.

Cellular detoxification and the subsequent rejuvenation is a great deal of work for each and every cell! That is why I advise those who are detoxing to AVOID working out. The body is in a constant state of labor, cleaning, eliminating, and rebuilding. It is tiring to say the least. While some may feel energized at first, it is not long until the incredible process of detoxification kicks in and fatigue of some sort ensues.

Low energy can also be a result of the cessation of coffee or other caffeine laden products that stimulate the adrenals into a false feeling of vitality.

Lastly, but extremely important is the understanding of animal protein and its effects on the body. I am often challenged with the concept that a detox participant feels "weak" with the removal of animal protein from the diet. They believe that animal protein somehow provides the body with "energy." It is carbon found in carbohydrates (sugar) that provides cells with energy to function, not protein. What animal protein provides (especially in the quantities consumed in the modern world) is addiction and adrenaline.

Just like coffee, sugar, salt, alcohol, or cigarettes are addicting, so too is animal flesh. The cessation of any of them can cause numerous symptoms, including fatigue. This occurs for many reasons, but foremost is the body working diligently to get rid of the stockpile of acid toxins that have built up over the years. Having the fortitude to push through and continue to detox will result in a very physical understanding that fruits and vegetables provide boundless amounts of energy and that animal protein will only serve to weigh the body down.

The sensation of increased energy that one may feel from eating a piece of steak or chicken can be explained by the ingestion of residual adrenaline found in the muscle tissue of the animal. As the animal is heading to slaughter, it has a sense of mortal danger from the procession of animals before him, each secreting oils from their anal glands as a response to absolute fear. This sends adrenaline rushing through the blood stream in a spontaneous fight or flight response. The job of adrenaline in this case is to increase heart rate, breathing, muscle response, pupil dilation, and allow the animal to fight or flee for its life. Of course, in this case, it can do neither and as the hammer comes down, the adrenaline is trapped in the animal's muscle tissue, unable to dissipate due to the act of slaughter. The muscle tissue gets butchered and shipped to grocery stores where it is purchased and then consumed. Thus, the receiver gets the protein, fat, iron, a few minerals, and a great deal of adrenaline. Therefore, taking animal flesh out of the diet is likened to removing coffee. The buzz, the kick, the "pick me up" is gone.

Should I stop detox?

No, low energy is temporary. Discontinuing detox is not the answer.

What to do.

Rest as much as possible, increase fruit consumption, and support the body and adrenal glands with the proper herbs.

Lung congestion

What it feels like.

Lung congestion may cause a feeling of tightness, pressure, or shortness of breath. There may be an expectoration of mucus or phlegm.

What it means.

This detox reaction can be a result of the release of toxins in a smoker or someone who has worked around toxic fumes, gases, smoke, or particles. It can also occur with someone who has a history of asthma, bronchitis, or pneumonia. These deep seated toxins are working their way out with the help of mucus and phlegm.

Should I stop detox?

Detox should not be stopped but can be slowed down for comfort. However, it is my belief that if you can handle the detox effects, then stay the course and dig deep!

What to do.

In traditional Chinese medicine, acupuncture followed by cupping is extremely helpful in breaking up congestion.

Lymphatic drainage massage as performed by a licensed massage therapist is also very beneficial.

Drink a cup of peppermint tea followed every 10 minutes with a half to a single teaspoon of the tincture of Lobelia (not to exceed five teaspoons). Lobelia is an antispasmodic at low doses and an emetic at higher doses. This could make an individual vomit. Vomiting will compress the lungs and expel the phlegm.

A castor oil pack with hot cayenne compresses, placed over the lung area on the chest or back, can also help to decongest phlegm followed by hot and cold compresses.

If lung congestion is coming on too strong you may introduce steamed vegetables or a baked sweet potato to slow down detox.

Swelling, itching, skin rashes, abscesses, oozing of pus

What it feels like.

These symptoms can be minute like a mosquito bite or intense like poison ivy. Skin symptoms can be brief, come and go, or last for days. The discomfort can range from a light itchiness to painful burning.

What it means.

The skin is the third kidney and a direct exit of waste, acid, and toxins out of the body. The process of detox opens all of the floodgates allowing the body to purge more easily. This can also be a sign of just how fatigued the kidneys have been, and now during the detox process, the skin is taking on some of the kidneys' work. It is also important to note where the skin issues occur. Rashes on the chest can relate to lung issues while rashes on the lower back can be related to the kidneys. If they occur on the extremities, then blood or lymph circulation can be the issue.

Should I stop detox?
No, this is a sure sign that you are moving lymph!

What to do.
DO NOT SUPPRESS. Allow the body to continue to eliminate. Support the body with appropriate herbs that will not only help the skin but also support kidney and bowel elimination.

Tepid baths with lavender oil, chamomile tea, Oregon grape root, Jamaican sarsaparilla, burdock root, bayberry root bark, white oak bark, and prickly ash bark are all supportive to the skin.

Lymphatic drainage massage, acupuncture, and cupping can all be beneficial.

Skin brushing (see resources).

Herbal healing salves (see resources).

Lemonade fast (see Chapter 13).

Weight loss

What it feels like.
Weight loss can mean various things to each individual. For most Americans, weight loss is a welcome side effect of detoxification. But for some, the loss of weight can actually be frightening. This is especially true for those individuals dealing with illnesses like thyroid disease, ulcerative colitis, or various forms of cancer. The emotional effects of weight loss can cause some individuals to believe

they are near death or dying. Others are caught in the social constructs connected to food, ranging from implications of anorexia to the latest psychological diagnosis of orthorexia (an obsession with eating foods that one considers healthy; a medical condition in which the sufferer systematically avoids specific foods in the belief that they are harmful).

What it means.

Weight loss means that the body is turning its attention to removing toxic matter as well as unnecessary tissue. The breakdown and subsequent removal of unnecessary tissue is known as *autolysis*—the destruction of a cell through the actions of its own enzymes. Each cell in the body contains the tools of its own destruction, and when we fast or significantly reduce dietary acid and calories, the body will break down nonessential substances for various reasons. Sometimes substances such as adipose (fat) are used for energy while other times the body chooses diseased tissue like benign or malignant tumors to break down and eliminate. But it does not stop there. The intelligence within the process of autolysis allows the body to get rid of unneeded tissue, while at the same time recycling aspects of that tissue for other purposes. For example, in the process of breaking down adipose cells, the body may recycle the fatty acids from those cells and use them as energy for muscles and other tissue. Adipose cells also synthesize and secrete complex fatty acid substances called prostanoids which carry out various hormone-like actions that can inhibit the breakdown of fat. They also synthesize a protein hormone called leptin, which helps in the process of regulating metabolism, body weight, and reproduction. These fatty acids and proteins are not destroyed, but recycled by the body and reused where necessary– after the process of autolysis. Therefore, when weight loss occurs during detoxification, even if the person is not overweight to begin with, it is not to be feared but understood and supported.

Should I stop detox?

This is a very important question and basically geared toward those who do not have excess weight to lose. When I began detox, I had previously lost 11 pounds in six days due to a thyroid storm. At 107 pounds I believed I was already at a deficit. The thought of losing another pound put me over the edge emotionally. But Dr. Morse assured me that it was "only weight" and promised that once my gut was clean and absorbing nutrition properly, my body would return to its normal weight, even on a detox diet. Sure enough, he was right, and by the time I finished detox I was back to the same weight I had been from age 19 to 44! That is not to say that I didn't go down to 99 pounds before recovery. But in the end, my body proved that it knew what it was doing and that it was capable of detoxification, healing, and regeneration!

So to answer the question, "should you stop detox?" the answer is generally no. I say generally because as I stated in previous questions, it is always good to work with a trained detox practitioner to analyze specific cases. That being said, I would not allow weight loss alone to halt the detox process.

What to do.

During detoxification one can find that they are deeply satisfied with the detox diet. Cravings vanish and energy is gained from a much smaller volume of food than what was consumed in the past. Frequently it is a challenge to convince them to eat more because they are quite satisfied with the amount of food they are consuming. But because the general population fears a certain number on the scale, and because the body is doing a great deal of work during detoxification, I recommend increasing calories in several ways.

1. Consume a larger volume of detox food.

2. Consume higher calorie detox foods such as avocados, bananas, dried fruits and baked sweet potatoes (yes, a 100% raw diet will generally yield a faster detox, but remember this is a marathon not a sprint and it is important to be able to sustain this process for the long haul for those who require a lengthy detox process).

3. Eat more frequently by nibbling throughout the day.

Other symptoms

MILD CLEANSING EFFECTS

1. Cold and flu-like symptoms

2. Low grade fevers (99-100 °F)

3. Coughing with or without discharge

4. Clear and yellow mucus discharge from nose or mouth (*this may include blood*)

5. Minor aches and pains

6. Mucus in stool

7. Mucus in urine

8. Loss of energy (may fluctuate)

9. Rashes and itches

10. Disease symptoms increasing temporarily

11. Mucus from eyes

12. Mild headaches

13. Minor blurred vision

14. Minor vertigo

15. Weight loss *(8–15 lbs. in two weeks. Depends on level of thyroid weakness. Can be as little as two pounds)*

16. Chills

17. Emotional feelings rising up, such as mild crying, anger or even laughter

18. Short term nose bleeds

19. Some rectal bleeding (*hemorrhoids or lesions*)

20. Minor blood in urine

MODERATE CLEANSING EFFECTS

1. Symptoms of bronchitis or pneumonia

2. Heavy discharge of green to brown mucus from nose and throat

3. Pain in joints

4. Heavy discharge from kidneys (*urine color changes to brown, orange, or dark yellow*)

5. Pain in old injuries

6. Minor paralysis of limbs

7. Chronic fatigue symptoms

8. Nose bleeds

9. Spasms of the lungs (*asthma/emphysema/C.O.P.D.)*

10. Moderate shortness of breath (*asthma/emphysema/C.O.P.D.*)

11. Temporary increase in tumor size

12. Disease symptoms magnifying (*short-lived*)

13. Sores appearing on the skin

14. Oozing of various substances from the skin, especially from the hands and feet

15. Bruising

16. *Weak* muscle breakdown (*muscle from meat protein*)

17. Heavy mucus discharge from eyes and ears

18. Vomiting

19. Diarrhea

20. Cellulitis "clumping"

21. Dizziness and/or vertigo

22. Minor heart palpitations

23. Loose teeth (*minor*)

24. Minor abscesses in mouth

25. Migraines

26. High-grade fever (103-105 °F)

27. Deep coughing (*sometimes dry*). Use herbs to loosen and eliminate (expectorate the impacted mucus

28. Depression or anxieties

29. Emotional releasing (*crying, anger, laughter, etc.*)

30. Heavy thoughts (*lack of clarity*)

31. Skin splitting

32. Excessive itching

33. Mercury tooth fillings can be pushed out of the body

34. Rectal bleeding from past or present hemorrhoids or lesions

I expect you to experience one, two, or more of these *healing crises symptoms*. While uncomfortable at times, there is no need to panic! These symptoms are a sure sign that your body is accepting the process of detoxification and working through it. It is proof that you are doing the program correctly and are benefiting from it.

Although this book is a guideline to detoxification and cellular rejuvenation, I strongly encourage you to work with a *qualified health care practitioner that has had advanced experience with detoxification and its side effects. Please see the Resource section at the end of this book.*

STRONG CLEANSING EFFECTS

1. Paralysis of any part of the body

2. Black mucus discharges from the lungs

3. Heavy brown discharge or blood in the urine with associated kidney pain

4. Heavy black discharge from the bowels with diarrhea

5. Tumors popping out all over the body

6. Loss of sight

7. Loss of hearing

8. Severe dizziness (*or vertigo*)

9. Severe fatigue

10. Abscesses of the mouth

11. Loss of fingernails or toenails

12. Excessive weight loss (*this can appear when a pancreatic weakness exists*)

13. Severe shortness of breath (*use an antispasmodic or inhaler*)

14. Temporary deep depression, released through crying, anger, laughter, etc.

15. Mental confusion

16. Skin cracking open

17. Teeth becoming loose (*major*)

18. Old suppressed symptoms (c.a. "poison ivy") reappear

Please keep in mind that most people do not experience the symptoms listed under **STRONG CLEANSING EFFECTS.** This is a very high level of detoxification. An individual's medical history, amount of stress, and degree of toxicity, as well as the strength or weakness of their genetic constitution will determine the intensity of a healing crisis. Those who are chronically ill or have a history of taking highly toxic or suppressant medications such as chemotherapy, radiation, prednisone, or anti-hypertensives can experience strong detoxification effects. The detoxification process may also cause a temporary flare in symptoms. Stay strong; know when to back off and consult a detoxification expert.

In regard to those that are taking multiple chemical medications, please DO NOT stop taking your medication *cold turkey*. Work with your health care practitioner to gradually wean yourself off of (or titrate) these potent medications. For example, as your blood pressure drops, your blood sugar normalizes, or thyroid numbers stabilize, it becomes clear that your body is recovering from a history of acidosis. Your doctor should be willing to lower current medication dosages to reflect your body's obvious and healthy improvements. If he or she is unwilling to work with you, it may be time to find a doctor who is open to the concept of disease reversal. As enticing as it may be to decrease your medication on your own, I do not recommend it. Continue to monitor all vital signs that pertain to your current medical condition(s).

Once again, I would like to emphasize, never fear a *healing crisis*, as these are as natural as breathing. Look at them as hurdles in a race. With each one you get closer and closer to the finish line!

Tell me something good!

When someone asks "Do you want to hear the good news or the bad news first?" I always choose the bad news. That being said, you have read all of the yucky physical and emotional things that can be experienced during detoxification. Now let's take a look at the light at the end of the tunnel.

Some of the most profound experiences my patients have when detoxing is an overall sense of well-being. This comes from two areas. First, it comes from making the decision to take control of your life and your health, and acting on it! You are no longer a passenger on a train, you are now the conductor! Second, there is an intoxicating feeling that one gains from raw, living food that is difficult to describe. Yes, you may experience some discomfort or a few healing crises, but there is a lightness of the body and mind that occurs from detoxification that is unrivaled by any other medical intervention. More specifically, bodily functions begin to stabilize.

Let's take a look:
1. Indigestion resolves

2. Headaches diminish and then resolve completely

3. Skin becomes brighter, rashes and acne disappear, while hair and nails become stronger

4. Dizziness resolves

5. Memory and focus improve

6. Energy increases

7. Blood pressure stabilizes

8. Blood sugar normalizes (by eating FRUIT!)

9. Breathing is eased as asthma symptoms vanish

10. Sinus congestion, post nasal drip, and allergies are eliminated

11. Tumors shrink

12. Moods improve

13. Menstrual cycle regulates and PMS resolves

14. Most menopause symptoms significantly reduce or resolve

15. Infertility resolves and pregnancy occurs!

16. Life is returned to the living!

These are just a handful of the astounding results of detoxification. I have detoxed people all over the world, and it never ceases to amaze me what the human body is capable of when it comes to healing. As you expand your health, I pray that in feeling better you will expand your capacity to love. Love is the only reason why we exist on this planet, and maybe if we felt better physically, maybe if we felt empowered, maybe if we felt a connection to ourselves again, we could learn to broaden our ability to love, to be loved, and to show love. The lack of love in the world today plays a tremendous role in why we get sick. If you are feeling unloved know this, I love you and more importantly you must love you! When you truly love yourself you can then cultivate the capacity to love others, which will in turn make you more lovable. Bring love into your detoxification process whether it be by affirmations, mantras, prayer, or just smiling in the mirror each day and your detoxification process will speed up exponentially.

Cultivating other healing practices
In Chapter 9: "Supportive treatment modalities," I discuss some of the natural therapies that can be incorporated into the detoxification process. But in this section, I would like to discuss some of the healing practices that you can perform on your own which will greatly improve your detoxification experience.

In our bi-monthly or monthly office visits, my patients share their experiences during detox as I question them regarding changes in their body. I have noticed that patients often feel they are not progressing until I review the intake form filled out during our first meeting. Initially, I asked questions about sleep patterns, body pains, energy level, digestion, and so on, as I took detailed notes of their responses. Four weeks later, when they are eager to share their personal accounts of healing crises, I ask if they notice any improvements. Many times the knee-jerk response is "I don't know." Then I pull out the original intake form. As we compare their current answers to those just four weeks prior, more often than not, there is improvement in many categories causing them to smile happily.

Sometimes it is difficult to see the positive changes, because as humans, we have a tendency to focus on the negative or what we perceive as negative (remember that a healing crisis is a POSITIVE effect of detox, not a negative one). Other times we may be scared to "get too excited" about the positive changes for fear of being let down. Keep in mind that many people have had health issues that are chronic, for which doctors have said there is no cure. I too, was afraid to admit that after just one week of detox, the tumor on my thyroid was actually shrinking! So I completely understand being hesitant about admitting progress. It is for this reason that I would like you to keep a journal.

Journaling

Keeping a journal will not cause you to wallow in the misery of illness. Instead, it will enable you to clearly monitor changes, crises, and improvements, while empowering you to continue on your healing journey. It will also serve as relevant documentation for your doctor or family members who challenge the process. It will provide you with clear evidence of your improvements while uncovering issues that you may not have known about, or show you just how your body reacts when you "cheat" on your detox diet. This is information that one cannot place a price on. It is invaluable. Your journal entries can be daily or every few days. If you have a superb memory, you can write a synopsis once a week, but please make sure that you document your journey.

Movement

As discussed earlier in this chapter, I am not an advocate of strenuous exercise during detoxification. My husband, Anthony, is an exercise enthusiast to say the least. He has been known to ride motocross, lift weights, work one on one with a personal trainer, run miles at a time, drag sandbags on the beach, and compete in obstacle course racing, all in one week. Prior to beginning detox, he was on a regimen of working out 1–2 times a day. Dr. Morse expressed to him that working out during detoxification was not only unhelpful, but in some cases detrimental. In Anthony's case, he was detoxing to resolve an issue of high blood pressure that had started three years prior. Following surgery to repair a fractured ankle (did I mention motocross?) his blood pressure increased and refused to come down to normal, even with acupuncture and Chinese herbs. But the diet and subsequent herbs which Dr. Morse prescribed resolved his hypertension completely within three short weeks. The detox process markedly decreased his energy levels, inhibiting him from working out twice a day, although he still managed a visit to the gym at least every three days. As I said before, detox uncovers underlying issues that you may not have been aware of. In Anthony's case, it uncovered an adrenal gland deficiency which shows up as *low blood pressure* causing him to feel weak and slightly light-headed. The anesthesia used during surgery acts as a neurotoxin causing a neurological type of hypertension. Once the toxins were cleared from his body, Anthony's "true" blood pressure was revealed. It was actually quite low due to an overwhelming amount of stress he had dealt with over the previous years between my illness and business issues. The good news was that now we were able to see his body clearly, and through several more months of detoxification and support to the adrenal glands, Anthony came back stronger than ever! His workouts continue to be epic and no feelings of weakness, light headedness, or hypertension have ever returned.

Through Anthony's story, I have emphasized the importance of limiting exercise during detox, but I do feel it is important for the body to move. Lying in bed or becoming a couch potato is not advised during detox either. After all, our emphasis in detoxification is to *move lymph!* As you have learned, lymph does not move on its own or with a pump (the heart) as blood does. Lymph moves due to the movement of your muscles squeezing and pumping lymphatic fluid and cellular waste as it makes its way out of the body via the kidneys, colon, and skin. There are several ways that you can keep the body happy and lymph moving while on detoxification. Here are some of my favorites:

- Walking

- Iyengar yoga

- Yin yoga

- Tai Qi

- Qi Gong

- Rebounding

- Swimming (a salt water pool or a body of fresh water is best)

- Jump rope

Movement is necessary to our lives. We are creatures that started off on this planet as nomads. Putting down roots in one spot has certainly served us in regards to building communities, but it has weakened us when it comes to understanding the incredible necessity the human body has for movement. Through detox and throughout life, keep moving!

Meditation/prayer/breath-work/thankfulness

These four words are subjects for hundreds of books in and of themselves, so the thought of me covering them in any type of depth is out of my realm of expertise. There are much wiser souls out there who have made it their life's work to tackle these topics superbly. Thus I encourage you to find a book, audio, or video recording that will appeal to you in one or more of these matters. However, I can address this subject in a broader view.

When I was struggling with the physical and emotional torment of Graves' disease, my anxiety had reached new heights. I was unable to sleep, focus, or concentrate. I felt abandoned by any higher power and I fought to keep my head above water, physically, emotionally, in my home life, and at work. I truly did not know which direction to turn when I received a phone call from an old friend. Gary was my former fire chief, fellow vegan (on and off), and overall good guy. He had heard that I was sick and called to see if there was anything he could do to help. I told him that I could not focus long enough to even come up with an adequate response and he said, I have an idea. A few hours later, he was at my door.

In the years prior to retirement, while Gary was still a fire chief, he was very interested in meditation. He had spent many years reading and studying about it although he did not actually meditate. He is an extremely analytical person and does not embark on anything without first researching it to death! Finally, after years of studying the scientific benefits of meditation as well as the vast variety of meditation practices, he began to focus on mindful meditation. His practice eventually lead him to participate in a 10 day silent meditation retreat called Vipassana. When he arrived at my house he was armed with a small cushion and a smile. Gary explained in simple terms the benefits of meditation and then took me through a short, delicately guided meditation that kept bringing me back to my breath. I felt my heart settle down and my muscles become more relaxed. He encouraged me to maintain a slight smile or grin while I followed my breath which gave me a feeling of hope. Unfortunately, I have not made time to participate in a 10 day Vipassana retreat, but it is on my bucket list. However, you do not have to separate yourself from your environment in order to separate your continuous thoughts from your body. Mindful meditation, guided meditation, prayer, breath-work, and taking time to be thankful for your life and the gifts that it brings (even illness) all provide you with the opportunity for growth, healing, and love of this life.

Community

One of the greatest struggles I encounter with my patients is the sense of being alone in this process. Rarely do family members, friends, or life partners embark on a detox protocol with them. Oftentimes they are mocked, teased, and constantly challenged about nutrition, starvation, and the never ending focus on protein (IF THIS HAPPENS TO YOU, PLEASE GIVE THEM A COPY OF THIS BOOK!). I recall Wayne Dyer once talking about the "tribe." He described the tribe as a group of people that you associate with. Whether they are family, friends, co-workers, or fellow members of a church, the tribe does not take well to change. Their fear of change spreads far past their own life and begins to seep into yours. They find comfort in the routine of life and even greater contentment if their level of stagnation extends to you. The tribe does not want to hurt you, but in their deep seated fear of change, they gravitate toward you and attempt to convince you that what you are doing "can't work; is crazy; keeps you from being social" or worse yet "is dangerous!" The tribe works harder to keep you "with them" than they would ever work to actually investigate or understand what you are doing. For that reason you must stay strong and learn to cultivate a like-minded community.

Cultivating a like-minded community is easier than you think. In fact, there may already be one out there! You can start close by, within the town or city that you live, or you can start far away, through social media. Since I prefer real people to virtual ones, I suggest that you begin in your own community.

The first step is to think about what kinds of people might be accepting to this type of detox process. A great place to begin could be in your local health food store. Look to see if there are workshops or lectures scheduled there that focus on natural healing, juicing, or cleansing. Granted, their cleansing process will likely differ from our detoxification program, but why not share what you know (and share my book) with others. You never know who YOU might help!

Next, try exploring the website **www.meetup.com**. This is a wonderful social organization which has created groups of people all over the world with vast interests, from dog walking to computer programming, not to mention vegan groups, raw food and detox groups, and juicing and exercise groups. You are bound to find one in your community that is welcoming of the path that you are on. And, if there is not one in your community yet, CREATE ONE!!! Yes, cultivate the community and support network that you desire in order to help yourself and to help others. After love, the next purpose we have on this planet is to help others. In the process you will help yourself and gain great success in Cultivating Unlimited Rejuvenating Energy! C.U.R.E. is what it is all about.

How long does it take?

I am often asked how long it will take to detoxify and reverse the process of disease in the human body. As much as I would like to answer this question with 100% accuracy, the truth is, it is just impossible to determine. Every single one of your 100 trillion cells has been through different experiences than every single one of my cells. Your genetic strengths and weaknesses, diet, life-style, stress levels, drugs, chemical exposures, and support system are all quite unique and therefore different from everyone else's. What you have in common is the absolute ability to remove acid waste, reduce inflammation, rebuild and restore cell function, and heal illness. How long that will take is unknown.

In my experience, there are several factors to acknowledge before attempting to draw a conclusion as to how long to detoxify. The detoxification process is anything but linear. There is an ebb and flow, if you will, to the process of healing. One day you feel like you are on the brink of recovery, and five days later, in the midst of another healing crisis. This natural phenomenon is not what we want in the fast-paced, instant gratification-based society that we live in, but it is the truth. And truth IS truth.

Factor #1: How long have you been sick and what is the severity of your illness?

How long you have been sick is preceded by how long it took you to get sick. Therefore, if you were diagnosed with high blood pressure two years ago, you can rest assured that the disease process was going on well over two years *before* the diagnosis. Adding on at least four years is a safe assumption. So there is a total of six years of acid build up that requires reversal. Does 21 days sound like an ample amount of time to reverse six years of acid? How about 42 days? 60 days? You get the picture. The disease process took quite a bit of time to build up in your arteries, to damage cells of the kidneys and weaken cells of the heart, all culminating into a neat packagecalled high blood pressure. This is a very important factor when determining how long to detoxify.

Also, how severe is the illness? Do you have abnormal cervical cells or have you been diagnosed with stage III cervical cancer? There is a difference. Yes, cells, blood, and lymph are all factors in both levels of the same illness. However, abnormal cervical cells are at the beginning stages of transformation compared to stage III. And remember, both issues began years before the diagnosis. Therefore there is a much deeper degree of acidity and lymphatic congestion that must be dug into in the stage III diagnosis.

Imagine that you live in the same house you lived in when you were born. Over time you received many objects, like diapers, clothes, toys and a bed. As you grew older you got books for school, pens, paper, and a backpack along with school clothes and sports accessories. Still older, you collected computers, cell phones, and a car. Along the way you ate food and drank liquids. Now imagine all of those things, including the wrappings that they came in, are still in your house. Everything you have ever owned is stacked, boxed, and tucked away in every nook and cranny. This is stage III cancer. This is Graves' disease with a thyroid storm. This is fibromyalgia with multiple sclerosis and rheumatoid arthritis. This is severe illness. This is not resolved by a 21-day juice fast.

Factor #2: Outside of acid food, what other lifestyle habits do you exhibit that are toxic and steal energy from the body?

When Cultivating Unlimited Rejuvenating Energy, we have to consider the conditions in life that draw energy from the body. In traditional Chinese medicine, each organ has its own energy or qi. The kidneys, for example, contain vital energy that I often describe as your body's bank account. Just like your financial bank account stores the money you make from working, the kidneys store vital energy that is gathered from good food, sufficient rest, and adequate physical activity. The goal of your financial bank account is to put a little more money in each month than what you take out. So too, the goal of kidney qi is to build a little bit more qi than what you expend. Expending kidney qi is done by overworking, over stressing, making poor food choices, and too much physical activity that is not balanced by adequate rest. When this happens, kidney qi becomes deficient, and imbalance and illness follow. On the flip-side, you can rebuild kidney qi or vital energy of the body by getting proper rest EVERY DAY, creating a fulfilling social life, managing stress with exercise, reading, yoga or meditation, and making proper food choices.

From a detoxification point of view, all of these things become factors in the ability of the body to detoxify efficiently, but there is more. Toxicity of the body is not drawn from acidic foods alone, it is also a result of the ingestion and inhalation of other substances. These include but are not limited to: tobacco in the form of cigarettes, cigars, pipes, chew and dip; marijuana, illicit drugs, prescription drugs and alcohol including wine; toxic fumes from various cars, trucks, buses and working around heavy machinery; jobs that expose you to dust from coal, other mined products, heavy metals; colorants, dyes and bleaches (such as in the salon industry); body care products such as toothpaste, deodorant, make up containing chemicals and metals such as mercury and aluminum; and chemical household cleaning products. All of these factors come into serious consideration when determining how long one might need to detox.

Factor #3: Stress
In all of the years I have been in practice and all of the people (including myself) that I have worked with, whether in acupuncture, homeopathy, or detoxification, I have rarely come across someone who does not complain of stress at some time in their lives. Mind you, stress has many faces and does not have to resemble Cameron Frye (Ferris' best friend) in "Ferris Bueller's Day Off!" Keep in mind that running or lifting weights is stress on your musculoskeletal system, but this is not a negative thing. Contemplating the holiday season can be stressful whether you have the perspective of Tigger the tiger (woo hoo!) or Eeyore the donkey (oh dear). The fact remains that a lifestyle devoid of downtime takes a large toll on your physical, mental, and emotional health and will hinder your body's ability to recover. Whatever the level or type of stress you have in your life, it is so very important that you find ways to manage it. The reduction and management of stress will propel your healing process to incredible heights.

Factor #4: The absence of symptoms is not the resolution of the problem.

My diagnosis came October 2010, followed by the thyroid storm in November 2010. I began to detox the last week of March 2011 and my blood tests all came back perfect by the end of July 2011. I finished my detoxification process March 2012. Yes, I detoxified for one year. Why did I choose to go for "so long" as many people might say? First, because I had a very severe illness as discussed in factor #1. Second, because the absence of symptoms or the improvement of numbers on a blood test is not evidence of cure. It is a good start, but not conclusive. I have, unfortunately, seen too many cancer cases where blood tests showed no sign of cancer markers or thyroid levels were "normal" only to "suddenly" go awry just a few months later because the patient insisted they were better and began to eat more acid-forming foods and discontinue herbs. Better, yes. Resolved, no.

That is not to say that detox must be ongoing for months or years without stopping. I actually stopped for 3–4 weeks around the seventh month. I gave myself a break, I "pulsed" off of herbs and still ate 100% clean and then jumped back in. Make no mistake about it, this detoxification process is for serious people with serious illnesses. It is for those with chronic conditions and acute infections. It is also for those who have a significant family history of a disease which they want to prevent. And serious illness, chronic conditions, acute infections and a history of disease in the family all require dedication and determination. Can I promise that an occasional pizza, brownie, or beer is not in your future during detox? Of course I cannot. We are modern humans after all with all of the temptations of modern times that wouldcertainly give Adam and Eve a run for their money! But have no fear. If you wander off the path, you are just a fruit smoothie away from getting back on track! Dig in and celebrate the return on your investment.

Factor #5: What do the eyes say? The science of iridology.
This topic can fill a chapter in and of itself. There are so many amazing books out there written by individuals who have studied the human iris to the nth degree that it is certainly worth doing some reading on the subject. For the

purpose of this chapter I will briefly address the subject of iridology as it has provided me with an observational tool that cannot be equaled in medicine.

In short, iridology is the study of the iris of the eye. The portion of the eye that shows the color. The iris is considered a "micro system" of the body much like the ear in Chinese medicine or the foot in reflexology. While the eye is the window to the soul, the iris is the tool that the creator gave us to allow us to see inside the body and determine its state of health. Within the iris we can observe one's physical history from birth to the present day. Also visible are genetic strengths and weaknesses, known as a person's constitution. We can also see chronic conditions and degeneration of tissues, organs, and glands, as well as the amount of lymphatic congestion, sulfa, sulfur and iodine that is stored in the body. Finally, the condition of the colon and digestive tract, as well as the brain and nervous system are all visible just by observing the iris. Iridology is a tool that naturopaths have used for hundreds of years. It continues to be a vital tool in the process of detoxification and can be a strong indicator of how long one must detoxify.

All of these factors come into play when determining the length of the detoxification process. It is as unique and individual as you are and it is my hope that by reading this book you will become an expert and inner physician of your body in order to create a process that will allow you to achieve C.U.R.E.

My advice to you is to begin this journey with the intention of detoxifying for at least six weeks. This is a short period of time in the grand scheme of things. With your journal and self-assessment questionnaire in hand, at the end of each week I would like you to read through your initial answers and the journal pages you have been keeping in order to evaluate your progress. This not only includes improvements (such as weight loss, lower blood pressure or decrease in body pain) but healing crisis (such as skin rashes, fatigue or headaches). With all that you have learned up until this point and the assessments made along the way, you will have a good idea whether to continue detox or ease off. As you move into your 6th week, decide what your next step will be. Will you continue on the path of detoxification or slow things down? What are you basing your decision on? How you are feeling? Emotions? Family pressure? It is important to know in your heart if your choice to discontinue the process is because you have achieved your personal health goals or is there another reason?

If you choose to stop detoxification after six weeks, I strongly recommend that you set a time in the future to delve in to detox again. Remember, if you have been on this planet for 20, 30, 40 or more years and have not eaten like the species that you are, there is much stagnant waste that needs to come out. Choose a time later in the year to embark on another six week (or longer) detox protocol.

On the other hand, if you evaluate your journal and the answers on your self-assessment questionnaire and determine that you are not finished, hoorah!!! Keep going! The deeper you dig into thedetoxification process whether it is through the length of time, the level of diet (see menus 1–3), or taking it up a notch with a lemonade or grape fast, please know that you are on a good path. This is a very sustainable process. As I mentioned earlier, I followed this detoxification for one year and till this day I remain on a diet that is 90% (or more) fruits and vegetables with that last 10% (or less) as nuts, seeds, oil and occasional grains like quinoa or brown rice or beans.

Please keep in mind that this process is dynamic and organic. It moves and changes with you and you must dig deep and tap into your inner self to truly reap the benefits. The relief of symptoms is passé and cloaked by allopathy. C.U.R.E. is truth and an awakening of the spirit; a knowing that it is no longer chained to a system that continues to tear it down and tear it apart. None of us are getting out of this alive. But in the time that we are here, we have the right to be healthy and happy. We have the right to have knowledge and truth and to be empowered by that truth. There is a time and a place for allopathy, but educate yourself as to when that is and take steps to care for your body in a more organic way.

The prevention of disease is far easier than the reversal of it. Even so, know that reversal is more than possible. Whether you are battling a severe illness, a mild ailment or you have no current health concerns, the process of detoxification should be undertaken by everyone more than once in a lifetime. Understanding the "cues" and "hints" that your body is giving you is enough to make the decision to detox. Headaches when you menstruate, sneezing after meals, stiffness upon waking or sensitivity to perfume are examples of hints your body gives to let you know there is lymphatic congestion. Do not allow T.V. commercials or magazine ads for heart burn or sinus congestion convince you that these issues are a normal part of being a human. They are not. Look inside your body in a different way. Iridology, traditional Chinese medicine pulse taking and tongue diagnosis or kinesiology testing are all ways to analyze the body's potential for a health issue long before an x-ray, CAT scan or blood test shows a problem.

"To ease another's heartache is to forget one's own."

- Abraham Lincoln

C | U | R | E *quotes*

chapter nine
Supportive Treatment Modalities

In the previous chapter I discussed the variables of how long one should detoxify. While there is not a universal timeline as to the duration of the detoxification process, there are supportive treatments and therapies that can be incorporated into your detoxification program. Such therapies will allow the body to detox more effectively, efficiently, and with greater ease. These treatments and therapies can also help to reduce the length and/or intensity of the healing crises as they occur. Please keep in mind that our intention is not to stop a healing crisis, but to support the body through it. Assistance through a healing crisis will ultimately keep you on course and allow you to obtain the healing results that you desire. This can only be accomplished if you stay the course. Impeding detoxification symptoms or healing crises is likened to what western medicine does on a regular basis by suppressing symptoms. Supportive therapies gently guide the body through the healing process, allowing the cells to purge their waste and coercing the eliminative organs to release waste to the outside world. These therapies support the building of new tissue by delivering vital blood, oxygen, nutrients, and energy (qi) to the cells while realigning the structure (bones, muscle, and connective tissue) so that blood and lymph can flow efficiently.

In this chapter I would like to introduce you to just a few of the supportive treatment modalities available, many of which I used during my own detoxification and healing process. I also provide various supportive modalities for my patients at Partners in Healing. These therapies have been around for hundreds to thousands of years, passed down from generation to generation. Their longevity is proof that they are both safe and extraordinarily effective. As an acupuncture physician, I have been asked many times, "Why did you not use solely traditional Chinese medicine (TCM) to heal your thyroid condition?" The answer is simple. 5,000 years ago, when TCM was being developed, there were no chemical antibacterial hand-wipes, no gasoline powered vehicles, no processed foods, no vaccinations, and no electronics. The advent of these acid-forming chemicals and electronics, though arguably helpful at times in modern life, has placed an enormous strain on our immune system and ultimately on our lymphatic system. While TCM is a remarkable form of natural therapy, it does not have the capacity to dig as deep as is necessary to C.U.R.E. and is just too limited in its spectrum of tools. The same can be said for chiropractic, massage therapy, sound therapy, and the like. However, when used in tandem with the detoxification and rejuvenation processes, these natural modalities are virtually unrivaled in their ability to reverse the process of disease and heal the body. Let's explore just a few of these supportive and natural treatment modalities.

Acupuncture and traditional Chinese medicine
TCM encompasses Chinese herbs, food therapy, qi gong (energy healing), tui na (Chinese massage therapy and body work), and of course acupuncture. These therapeutic modalities have been used for nearly 5,000 years and are documented in numerous books, the oldest of which dates back to 2697 AD. There is virtually no ailment or illness that cannot benefit from TCM, whether it be acute or chronic pain from trauma, functional issues such as irritable bowel disease or asthma, or hormonal issues such as infertility or diabetes.

While ancient texts do not refer to these disorders by their modern Western medicine names, they are described in such great detail that it is remarkably simple for one to deduce what disorder TCM is referring to. The only significant difference is the name of the disorder. For example, in TCM diabetes is known as either a lung, stomach, or kidney yin deficiency. Therefore, the treatment would be to choose acupuncture points and Chinese herbs that would nourish "yin," or fluids of either lung, stomach, or kidney. Food therapy would also be used, keeping in mind that processed foods would never be recommended and observation of the patient's symptoms (including tongue and pulse) would be the gauge used to determine if the treatment is working effectively. As stated earlier, TCM is not capable of reversing ailments such as diabetes or Graves' disease, as the level of toxicity in modern times is so great that ancient traditions fall terribly short. In fact, the levels of toxicity in modern life were virtually unheard of thousands of years ago. This is where detoxification comes in, to take the body's ability to heal itself to the next level.

When it comes to detoxification, support is where TCM prevails. There are numerous issues which can benefit from treatments like acupuncture, Tui Na, and qi gong during the process of detoxification. I'll list a few of the foremost issues below and describe just a few reasons to incorporate TCM into your detoxification process.

1. Side effects or healing crises: Acupuncture has an uncanny ability to deal with pain, especially when old pains are reawakened by detox. Acupuncture will not cover up pain but allow the body to work through it more rapidly. It will also be quite effective in moving past nausea, headaches, abdominal discomfort, and fever due to detox.

2. Stress, anxiety, and mood swings may also occur during detoxification and also benefit from acupuncture.

3. Food cravings: These will self-resolve within the first 2–3 weeks of detoxification. But in the beginning when you are just getting your "fruit" legs, acupuncture can really help control those mental or physical cravings.

4. TCM can increase the speed at which swellings, inflammation, and growths diminish.

5. Sinus, nasal, and lung congestion. Acupuncture can open up these areas quickly allowing breathing to occur more effortlessly. The effects of this process are not short-term, but long lasting. Acupuncture benefits can persist for hours or even days after a treatment.

6. Support of the eliminative systems, the kidneys, colon and skin. It is well known that during detoxification several systems get pushed to their limits. As acid waste is dumped

from the cells into the lymphatic system, these symptoms may occur.

- Burning upon urination. This resembles a urinary tract infection, but it is not. The use of acupuncture can quickly and effectively mitigate this symptom, strengthening kidney function and reestablishing harmony of the tissues.

- Diarrhea. This can be a result of increased fiber in the diet along with detox herbs. Usually one or two acupuncture treatments will resolve this symptom.

- Constipation can be a result of acid waste dumping into an already overloaded colon. Even if you have less than 1–2 bowel movements a day prior to detox, it is imperative to use supportive herbs for the stomach and bowels so that they can keep up with the increased work load. Acupuncture is superb at aiding these eliminative processes.

- Lack of sweat. For various reasons including endocrine issues (primarily thyroid and adrenal glands) and severe lymphatic congestion, the body can fail to eliminate waste via the skin. If this occurs, TCM has very specific acupuncture or pressure points that can induce sweating.

There are many other benefits to TCM during and after detoxification. The question of how often or how many treatments are necessary is up to the individual, their detox effects, their body's response to acupuncture, and a frank discussion with your A.P. During my detoxification, I was blessed to have a very dear friend and fellow A.P. treat me 1–2 times a week for a month or so. As my body began to improve and healing crises decreased, I was able to reduce my treatments to 1–2 times a month. Once you have completed your detox process it is always a good idea to see your A.P. for a "tune-up" at least four times a year.

Chiropractic

Chiropractic is a system of natural therapy based on the diagnosis and subsequent manipulative treatment of misaligned joints, especially those of the spinal column. These misalignments contribute to physical disorders of the body by affecting the nerves, muscles, and organs. Chiropractic manipulation is a very important part of ensuring the most natural movement and function of the body as possible. While chiropractic is said to be a little older than 100 years (founded in 1895 by Daniel David Palmer), its roots reach back to osteopathic physicians, naturopathic physicians, and even as far back as 2700 AD in ancient Greece. This therapy is yet another natural treatment with no serious side effects and tremendous benefits.

During my detoxification process, my body went through a great deal of pain. Initially the pain was related to the enormous amount of muscle tension due to the stress of the disease and all of the issues that accompanied it. Severe muscle tension can ultimately tug at spinal bones, known as vertebrae, pulling them out of alignment, which can lead to more pain as well as impingement of nerves.

Another aspect connected with having chiropractic adjustments during detoxification is the feeling of being in a supportive environment. Although my chiropractor (who is also a co-worker) knew nothing about this detox prior to my illness, he was trained to view the human body in a very holistic fashion. His willingness to listen, discuss, and understand the process of detoxification allowed me to feel supported in a much deeper way. Together, we discovered the changes that detox made to my body and the adjustments that he could make to aid those changes. I underwent adjustments weekly for the first two months of detox, after which I tapered off and only had adjustments as needed.

Cranial Sacral Therapy (CST)

CST is a gentle, hands-on method of evaluating and enhancing the function of a physiological body system called the craniosacral system—comprised of the membranes and cerebrospinal fluid that surround and protect the brain and spinal cord. CST is performed by a licensed massage therapist, acupuncture physician, or chiropractor who has been trained (traditionally by The Upledger Institute) to feel blockages of the rhythmic flow of cerebral spinal fluid as it circulates through and around the brain and spinal cord. With patience and a delicate touch, the therapist releases these blockages allowing the body to reestablish a homeostatic balance. This release will also enhance the purging of toxins from the brain's lymphatic system (known as the glymphatic system) into the larger lymph system for removal via the kidneys, colon, and skin.

CST is one of the most remarkable therapies that I have ever experienced. After falling from my horse and fracturing my pelvis three years prior to having Graves', CST was the only treatment able to help me fall asleep during and after my stay in the hospital. I was in such terrible pain, that even the most powerful medication was not able to allow me to rest. Luckily I had a dear friend, Laura, who came to the hospital and treated me. Since CST does not require one to disrobe or lie on the abdomen, she was able to softly slide her hand under the sheet and apply the gentlest pressure to my sacrum, mid back, and occiput. I honestly do not remember her leaving the room after that first session. I fell asleep for the first time in three days just from her touch.

One of the most compelling effects of CST was during my detoxification. Along with the diagnosis of Graves' disease, I had an enlarged thyroid known as a goiter. As you learned in previous chapters, a tumor or enlarged gland is a result of acid toxins congesting the lymphatic system causing the cells to become inflamed, deteriorate, or become deformed and malfunction. During my third CST session, the therapist noticed an obvious reduction in the size of the goiter. We were both stunned by the changes that occurred even *during* therapy. Moreover, the effects of CST were not fleeting, they were lasting. In the end, we felt that the goiter would not have vanished that rapidly with detox alone. CST, like acupuncture, TCM, and chiropractic, sped up the healing process allowing the alkaline diet and therapeutic herbs to work much more efficiently and effectively in my body.

I highly recommend CST as a supportive therapy through detoxification as well as an important tool for maintaining optimal health. As a practitioner of acupuncture and natural therapies, I am hard pressed to find another hands-on modality that produces greater results than CST when treating physical trauma and cellular imbalance. Please see Chapter 14: "Recipes and Resources" for more information.

Lymphatic Drainage Massage

Lymphatic drainage massage, also called lymphatic drainage therapy or manual lymph drainage (MLD) is a technique developed in Germany for treatment of lymphedema, an accumulation of lymphatic fluid that can occur after lymph nodes are surgically removed. Most often lymph nodes are removed after a mastectomy as a result of breast cancer, although any cancer surgery can prompt their removal as well. Lymphedema can also occur without the removal of lymph nodes. This is due to acid toxicity and the buildup of waste within the lymphatic fluid between the cells (interstitial space).

When one or more lymph nodes are removed from a person's body it is likened to disconnecting the septic tank from a house. As you recall in Chapter 2: "The Science of Sickness," the septic tank collects all of the waste that comes from the sinks, bath tubs, showers, and toilets in the house. Once the waste is deposited into the septic tank, numerous bacteria get to work at breaking the raw waste down. This is known as sewerage. As more waste and water enters into the septic tank, older, more processed sewerage gets pushed out into a drain field. This allows the sewerage to slowly get absorbed into the ground. If the septic tank were removed, the pipes leading from the sinks, showers, tubs, and toilets would dump directly into the ground surrounding the house. As you imagine, this causes a mass flood of waste water seeping up from the ground. The end result is smelly, saturated earth encompassing your home like a moat, attracting bugs, parasites, and the like.

While the thought of removing a septic tank sounds ludicrous as well as disgusting, so too is the removal of lymph nodes. The extrication of lymph nodes from the body leaves the patient with an incomplete lymphatic system, resulting in swelling of the arms and/or legs. That swelling is lymph fluid which is filled with acidic cellular waste. The fluid collects around the cells, rapidly creating an acidic environment leading to inflammation, disease, and eventual cell death. That is where manual lymphatic drainage massage comes in.

While I do not advocate the removal of lymph nodes, if the damage has been done, then manual lymphatic drainage along with detoxification is the knight in shining armor. Almost before my eyes, I have witnessed amazing changes in the reduction of swelling and inflammation. This very, very light touch is life giving and miraculous and should be an essential therapy offered in every surgeon's office. A protocol of MLD should be implemented after every surgery regardless of lymph node removal, but certainly if they have been removed. Toxic anesthesia can be assisted out of the body along with dead cells caused by traumatic injury that is by definition, surgery.

However, this is a book about detoxification and you've likely not had lymph nodes removed, nor undergone surgery. What could MLD do for you? As the title of this chapter states, MLD is yet another valuable therapy that supports the detoxification process. How so? As your body goes through detoxification, a heavy load is placed on the eliminative systems of the body (kidneys, colon, and skin). However, prior to elimination of waste to the outside world, the lymphatic system is greatly taxed. As cells are encouraged to dump their waste into an already toxic lymphatic system, symptoms can arise. Oftentimes there is pain in the muscles and/or joints. In other cases, swelling of appendages, pressure, or congestion in the head and lungs, headaches and even dizziness can occur. MLD can help in all of these cases.

MLD is achieved with the lightest of touches so as not to inflict more pain or discomfort to the body, but instead to gently guide the lymph into appropriate lymph vessels, to the nodes and then to the eliminative systems. This is a soothing and relaxing therapy that can be incorporated after 1–2 weeks of detoxification. I prefer my patients to have one or two weeks of an alkaline diet and herbs under their belt before starting MLD. This allows alkaline food and astringent herbs to begin the process of breaking up and loosening congestion. At that point, MLD 1–2 times a week is very effective.

Of course it is highly recommended that you find a licensed massage therapist that is certified in MLD. Please see the resource section to help located a therapist near you.

Sound, Vibration, Color and Light Therapy

I prefer to group these therapies together as the practitioners that I have worked with in my office frequently combine these in one treatment session. During my own detoxification process, I became the patient of another very dear friend and fellow acupuncture physician. She specializes in what is known as *Acutonics,* a form of sound and vibrational therapy. "Sound therapy" utilizes tuning forks as does Acutonics, the main difference being what the instruments are "tuned" to. In Acutonics, the forks are tuned to the vibrations of the planets within our solar system. In sound therapy, they are tuned to the musical notes which we are all familiar with. I cannot say that one is superior to the other. They are different and it is up to the individual to decide which one resonates with them. I love them both! Allow me to share some information about this unique, yet age old therapy.

Sound is older than the spoken word. Before language there was sound. Wind blowing through the trees, birds chirping, animals communicating, and rivers cutting through rock, dirt and foliage while volcanos erupted and storms surged, creating the sounds and vibrations of life. The resonating sounds traveled miles and miles, affecting the masses they came in contact with.

The human body has its own rhythmic patterns. The beating of the heart, rhythmic pulsations of cerebral spinal fluid, movement of lymph and continuous neurological sparks are all examples of the vibrational melody of our remarkable human bodies. As science continues to study quantum physics, there is growing evidence that the rhythms of the heart, brain, and other organs enjoy a special synchronicity that cannot yet be understood by modern medicine. Much like energy blockages of the meridian system in traditional Chinese medicine, it is believed that illness can arise when these inner rhythms are disturbed.

Sound therapy, which includes tuning forks, singing bowls, chimes, of sounds and vibrations to induce change in the body on a physical, emotional, and cellular level. Whether the sound is traveling through the body or being listened to, the specific instrument or tone used can create numerous body balancing and cellular healing responses. Sound therapy affects many aspects of the body from pain relief and activating meridian systems, to supporting physical detoxification and the release of negative mental and emotional holding patterns. This is a full body treatment, providing holistic healing in all realms, including physical, mental, emotional, and spiritual imbalances.

Color Light Therapy induces change in the body on a cellular and emotional level. Light exists as both waves (which we can see) and photons (particles); the latter enter the brain and body via the eyes and the skin to initiate response on a cellular level.

Emotional Freedom Technique (EFT)
I first learned of EFT about 10 years ago, when I was signing up for some continuing education courses. I had never heard of it before, but the class was offered in a quaint city in Florida, just a few hours north of where I lived, so I combined CEU's with a visit to a warm mineral spring. What I learned that day was truly profound and has helped me through some tough times.

Emotional Freedom Techniques, or EFT (often known as Tapping or EFT Tapping), is a universal healing tool that can provide impressive results for physical, emotional, and performance issues. EFT operates on the premise that no matter what part of your life needs improvement, there are unresolved emotional issues in the way. Even for physical issues, chronic pain, or diagnosed conditions, it is common knowledge that any kind of emotional stress can impede the natural healing potential of the human body.

EFT combines the physical benefits of acupuncture with the cognitive benefits of conventional therapy without the use of needles. Instead EFT relies upon a unique process of tapping particular acupuncture points in a specific order. In many cases, the results are a much faster, more complete treatment of emotional issues, and faster resolution of physical and performance issues compared to acupuncture alone.

*"These pains you feel are messengers.
Listen to them."*

- Rumi, The Essential Rumi

CURE *quotes*

chapter ten
Consciousness

I have worked in various areas of the healthcare industry over the last three decades. In my early 20's I was a fitness instructor and personal trainer. From my mid 20's to late 30's I changed professions and worked as a firefighter/EMT, and over the past 14+ years I have been in practice as an acupuncture physician (A.P.). In each of these professions, I have dealt with people who struggle with their health and weight. They were firmly seated on the dieting roller coaster, looping around and around, in and out of fad diets, around the latest food novelties and through prescription or over-the-counter medical trends. They rarely reached their goal weight and were rarely able to maintain it if they did.

As the owner of an aerobic studio, I often counseled clients on the basics of the 'calories in- calories out' theory. We talked about reducing fat and calories while increasing exercise. As firefighters we were required to have yearly physicals which restricted some firefighters to "light duty" due to their weight-induced hypertension, diabetes, or heart disease. In my current practice I have often been asked if acupuncture needles can help someone eliminate hunger or stop eating.

When I recall conversations I have had with people struggling to lose weight, there is one piece in the puzzle I understand now that I did not truly understand then…unless you bring consciousness into the realm of food, nutrition, and eating, you will forever be chasing a diet mirage. The lack of consciousness is the root of all that is wrong with our relationship with food and our health. Without it, we are destined to loop around and around on the roller coaster, never able to get a grip on our health or our weight.

So what is consciousness? What role does it play in body fat or autoimmune disease? How does being conscious contribute to happiness and optimal health, while the lack of it influences immune function or cancer? And how do I attain it? For me, consciousness is a state of tapping into truth; removing myself from a state of denial while bringing awareness to myself. There is a reason why we eat the "wrong" food, too much food, or maybe not enough food and there is no pill to fix it. Only consciousness will free us from this struggle.

There is an idiom about burying your head in the sand. To me, this is the essence of being unconscious. You know that there is something out there, something that is just around the corner; just on the other side, out of our sight. But it may be too painful to look at, too difficult to face. Yet the pain and suffering that we experience by not facing the truth is ultimately far worse than the pain of coping with it.

Before I was diagnosed with Graves' disease, I knew that I was pushing myself relentlessly. I worked 48 hours a week as a firefighter while obtaining my bachelor and then master's degree. After graduation, I continued to work as a firefighter while I built my acupuncture practice. Once I left the fire department and became a full time acupuncture physician, I learned the harmful art of *always saying "yes."* My patients were busy people and could not always make it to their appointments during my scheduled office hours. So of course, I would accommodate and come in early (7 a.m.) or stay late (I have been in my office as late as 9 p.m. in the past). All the while I ignored the consciousness that could have saved me from myself. The pain and suffering I experienced during the thyroid storm, along with the humiliation I felt when the doctor asked if I ever noticed the large goiter on my throat was enough to finally wake me up! That was the impetus into consciousness.

A Lesson in Consciousness

In the modern world one might deduce that wild animals exhibit more conscious awareness than humans do. They are keenly aware of their surroundings, making sure they are as safe and comfortable as possible. This is not only important for animals, it is equally important for humans as well. Your first lesson in consciousness is to become aware of your environment. Where are you sitting while you read this book? Are you in a chair, on the sofa, or in bed? Is the surface under your rear end firm or soft? How is the lighting? Is the TV on? Are you alone or are there others around? What is the ambient temperature? Are you comfortable? After all, you paid good money for this book. Wouldn't you want to set yourself up to get the very most out of it?

This is the first step into consciousness, becoming aware of the environment around you. Once aware, you can choose to keep the environment as it is or change it. Turn on another light. Turn off the TV or go to another room completely. If that is not an option perhaps you might decide to read in your car. Whatever changes you make, you are making them consciously. You are choosing to make this reading experience the best it can be in order to gain the most that you can from it.

Now let us take this lesson in consciousness a step further. In order to do so, I would like you to gather a few things. If you have to put the book down to get them and then return, I can wait. I would like you to go to your pantry or the grocery store and obtain a box of Saltine Crackers (or the gluten-free equivalent if you are allergic or sensitive to gluten) and a package of fresh organic strawberries, grapes, or a watermelon. Whichever you prefer.

Now that you have your tools for this lesson, here are your directions:
1. Take out a single cracker and take a substantial bite. Did you feel resistance or did the cracker crumble easily between your teeth? Chew very slowly noticing the texture, dryness and saltiness of the cracker. Was the taste flavorful or flat? Pay attention to the sensation of the cracker as you begin to swallow. How does it feel against your palate, the back of your throat and into your esophagus? What do you experience from incorporating that cracker into your body? Do you feel nourished, nurtured, satisfied or energized? Or do you feel weighed down or empty?

2. Now take the fresh strawberry, grape, or chunk of melon. Bite into it with your front teeth. Did you notice any resistance? Was there a firmness followed by a softness? Did it feel sticky, juicy, wet, or dry? Did you just taste sweetness or was there a tartness, tanginess, or bitterness to the bite? What is going on inside of your mouth? Do you feel the release of saliva? Is there more fluid around your tongue? As you chew, does the taste continue to blossom or become dull? Now swallow and notice if the fruit moved down your throat with ease or resistance? Finally how do you feel? Are you energized? Do you feel nurtured or nourished?

This is a simple exercise that teaches you how to be mindful when eating. Becoming mindful of the consumption of your food allows you to "ask" your cells if they are happy with your choice of food or not. Allow me to elaborate.

I am sure you have heard of or used the phrase "gut feeling" or "gut instinct." This term, while used indiscriminately, truly explains the consciousness of each and every cell in our bodies. Animals are acutely in touch with their gut instinct. If you watch a dog or cat when approached by a person who does not particularly care for animals or exhibits aggressive body language, the animal will respond with aggression or fear. When you meet someone for the first time, it is common to have an immediate "feeling" about them. You may either resonate with their personality, soul, or being, or you may not. I am not saying that you either love or hate them in an instant, but you get a sense of drawing closer or pulling back. This is the essence of gut feelings. In relation to food, if you take the time to touch, taste, and feel your food within you, and then go a step further to "ask" your body if this food is a positive choice for you or not, you will get an answer. In the gut! This is the level of consciousness that we are innately blessed with for our survival.

Finally, let's tap deeper into understanding consciousness by exploring our internal environment. You remember, don't you? Your body and how it feels. I'm not necessarily talking about how you feel when you have an illness, ailment, or a diagnosis. I am talking about how you feel on a regular basis. Do you wake up in the morning without an alarm clock or do you have to have some form of outside stimulus prompting you to start your day? Do you feel stiff or achy when you get out of bed? Or are you spry and quick to move? Do you wish that you could just stay in bed a little bit longer or hope that it is the weekend and your alarm clock went off accidentally? Do you have a headache or a stuffy nose? Or do you immediately trudge off to the kitchen robotically, reaching for that first cup of coffee? Are you even consciously aware of these things? Tapping into consciousness once again, I want you to really analyze yourself. Ask yourself whether you wake up tired, achy, and in need of caffeine in order to be able to start your day. Then ask yourself if you believe this is healthy, normal, or good for you.

When we tap into consciousness instead of following a mindless routine, we become markedly aware that we don't feel well. We begin to realize that reliance on a stimulant or waking up with a headache is not normal (even if common), and more importantly, a sign that something more serious is going on. We realize that these symptoms are a plea for help from every cell of our body. Conscious awareness allows us to make an observation about our life and then make a conscious effort to change it. Without consciousness, we will continue to go through life believing that the fatigue, aches, pains, illnesses, and diagnoses that we receive are a normal part of life or getting older. We remove the responsibility from ourselves and believe that we have no control. Worse yet, we live in such a cloud of disconnect that we do not even realize that we feel poorly. So we continue to reach for that 2nd or 3rd cup of coffee, Tylenol, a heating pad, nasal spray or blood pressure medication, mindlessly trudging through our day.

Without consciousness, the human body falls into deeper and deeper disarray, making it more and more difficult to climb out. The effort that it would take to change after 40, 50, or 60 years of living this way can feel insurmountable, leaving us with the choice of staying in our walking coma, or challenging our status quo and being uncomfortable for a period of time. But the discomfort of becoming conscious and making healthy life changes is nowhere near the detriment of letting an unhealthy lifestyle persist.

I had a patient, "Jennifer," some years ago that came to me with digestive issues. She was a very sweet woman who chose nursing as her profession. Jennifer dealt with chronic indigestion, belching, heart burn, and difficulty swallowing for nearly two years. As with many people, she took over the counter and prescription medications, but her condition continued to worsen. She had heard about the detoxification program that I do with my patients from a nurse that she worked with and was interested in trying it. After a two hour consultation with me, she embarked on the alkaline diet and herbal protocol, specifically tailored to her needs.

Over the next four weeks, each time she came to the office, we discussed her symptoms, how closely she was adhering to the program, and her progress. To my dismay, she was not improving. While she followed the alkaline diet only about 80% and took all of her herbs I expected to see some amount of improvement as digestive issues tend to resolve quite quickly on this program. By the fifth week, I advised her to see a medical doctor and have an endoscopy done. She balked for a few moments but finally relented. One week later, we had the results–esophagus cancer. She was devastated and confided in me that the doctors convinced her to do chemotherapy much to her apprehension. She wanted to remain on the detox program to provide much needed support through such a toxic therapy. I agreed to continue to work with her as she went through chemotherapy.

Two days later she called me with new found empowerment! "F**k them," she shouted! "What was I thinking?" "I don't believe in any of that crap!" She had decided to follow the detox protocol 100% and forgo chemotherapy completely. That is a very personal decision and I would never ask a patient to make that choice. But she never believed in chemo in the first place and even though I was willing to support her through it, she chose to follow the path of consciousness.

Over the next seven months she worked diligently at the process. It was challenging, and there were many weeks where she could only get fresh-pressed grape juice down her throat due to the obstruction. But she persevered and we celebrated her success when she could finally eat a salad with little discomfort. Unfortunately our celebration was short lived. She wandered away from the program seeking out other "natural" forms of therapy, at times going completely to the acid side of chemistry.

Consciousness means staying in the moment. Understanding your successes, as small as they may seem, and persevering. Our unconscious mind, the one that may not acknowledge the tremendous shift from not swallowing to swallowing, seeks comfort in sedation. To sedate our senses with mind numbing non-foods like canned, creamy soup or Oreo cookies takes us away from the consciousness of real food gliding down the throat, unobstructed.

The tumor returned and eventually overtook her. Consciousness in regard to changes in the body are extremely important. Changes can be slight or massive signs, communicating from the physical body to the mental body to pay attention. They warn us that something is wrong and beg us to take care of it before it gets worse. Those little, seemingly insignificant nuisances that prompt us to reach for a TUMS, an aspirin, or coffee are warning us of future trials and tribulations. Only if we are conscious can we truly be proactive in our health and engage in prevention.

We have talked about conscious awareness of your external environment and how it affects you. We have acknowledged that being in touch with your physical body and how you feel is extremely important to gauge whether the body is on its way to disease and illness. In addition, we have talked about being conscious on a cellular level and how your food directly affects every cell in your body. Lastly I would like to discuss consciousness in relationship to your thoughts and their effect on your health. In one of her books, the author Marianne Williamson talks about our thoughts and their ability to bring us to "heaven or hell." Reading that had a very profound effect on me and caused me to monitor my thoughts far more closely than ever before.

Consciousness begins in our mind and with our thoughts. We can choose to be aware of how food affects us or not. Either way, it is our thoughts that first bring us to that awareness. But let's go deeper. Our thoughts about which food will best nourish us can then manifest as physical action by choosing to eat nourishing food. So our conscious choice to eat a bowl of grapes leads to a positive physical outcome. But, how do our thoughts alone lead to a positive or negative outcome in our body? What is the physical connection between our mind and our body, and how does it affect our health?

One of the best analogies I can give you is a famous children's cartoon character. He is a dear friend of Winnie the Pooh and his name is Eeyore the donkey. Eeyore is characterized as a pessimistic, gloomy, and depressed stuffed donkey who seems incapable of experiencing pleasure. Eeyore always sees the dark side of life and it seems he cannot get out of his own way when it comes to his negative thoughts. As Eeyore expresses his feelings, his body language mirrors his emotions. And as we watch Eeyore, we can't help but feel sad, discontent, or hopeless. This cartoon character's energy actually has an effect on our energy! Contrast Eeyore's persona with Tigger the Tiger. It is impossible not to smile when Tigger comes bouncing into the room! He brightens the day and makes us feel giddy! Again, this is a cartoon, yet it has a profound effect on the viewer.

Next notice how your thoughts about those two characters affect you. You are not even watching the cartoon and yet you frown or smile, smirk or grimace at the thought of the characters. Finally, consider your thoughts concerning your personal life, the news you watch, or your anticipation of an upcoming festive event. How do these thoughts make you feel? How do words expressed by a newscaster, the greeting in a birthday card, or an argument with a friend affect you physically? Do you feel things in your chest or your gut? All of these examples have to do with energy and vibration.

Thoughts, positive or negative, have a direct energetic effect on the body which is expressed through vibration. Remember a few paragraphs ago when I mentioned meeting someone for the first time and feeling a resonance with that person? You are drawn to them or repulsed. What occurs in your body when your thoughts or feelings take you somewhere?

On a cellular level the vibration that occurs is similar to tapping the ends of a tuning fork together, but on a much more delicate level. It can be prompted via neurotransmitters released by the adrenal glands. A scary experience, like losing control of your car for several seconds on a busy highway, prompts an immediate response by the adrenal glands. Adrenaline is released into the blood stream triggering a cascade of reactions in the body. Pupils dilate, heart rate increases, blood pressure elevates, breathing becomes shallow and rapid, and the muscles of the extremities become engorged with blood, leading to a feeling of muscular tension. This is what is known as fight or flight. Long term chronic stress in life continuously causing this fight or flight response can ultimately lead to a weakened immune system, erratic blood pressure, chronic muscle pains, or hormonal imbalances, to name just a few. The most interesting thing about the fight or flight response is not that it occurs automatically when we are threatened, but that it occurs when we *think* about being threatened. Mentally recounting an argument with a friend or recalling a car accident you were involved in can elicit the same physical response in the body as actually being in the situation. Therefore, your thoughts directly influence your body and your health!

Consciousness in your daily life, from what you choose to eat, to how you choose to think about or perceive life, has an absolute effect on your health. This is an extremely empowering concept that stands to cause profound changes in your body! While some may look at consciousness as a lot of work, I challenge you to see it as freedom. Consciousness is freedom to create, develop, and travel through your life the way YOU want to. You are no longer a sheep, following the herd. You now have a deep stake in the game of life! Of course, I realize that I do not have control over every aspect of life and as the saying goes, sometimes "sh** happens." Or as my husband likes to say, "man plans and God laughs!" The truth of the matter is, once you step into the world of consciousness, you have empowered yourself with a much more active role in your fate.

Incorporating Consciousness into Life
As stated previously in this chapter, there are many ways to work toward consciousness. Becoming aware of the environment around you, whether it be the thermostat in your house, the bed you sleep in, or the company that you keep. Begin to make conscious choices that

will improve your existence. That doesn't mean spending gobs of money on a fancy new car. Quite the contrary. Maybe it means spending less on a car payment so that you can do more in your life like travel, plan dinners with loved ones, or donating to charity. Perhaps choosing a poignant documentary instead of another grisly terrorist movie. The point is, make conscious choices and not impulse decisions in your life, and you will find that you feel much more content.

When making dietary choices, we can look at food in several ways.

1. Is it feeding a nutritional need?

2. Is it feeding an emotional need?

3. Is it feeling a craving?

4. Can it feed all three?

How great would it be if your conscious choices in food could feed all needs from nutrition to taste, to that warm fuzzy comfort that we as humans get from our food? The truth is that it can! We can have flavor, nutrition, and JOY in our diet! When we make a choice to eat consciously, it is almost impossible to make poor food choices. And if we do make that choice for a New York style pizza, the good news is that we made it with awareness and we should revel in that choice!

Many years ago, my cousin Mary and I made a pact to visit each other every two months. We live about four and a half hours apart, so every other month, one of us would drive to the other's house for a long weekend. We always had a great time whether she came to Fort Lauderdale or I went to Tampa. But I must admit, I thoroughly enjoyed my visits to Tampa more! You see, before I became vegan, we had a ritual. I would arrive at her house around 3:00 p.m. on a Friday. Mary would help me unload my belongings from the car which included a small suitcase, cosmetics, blow dryer bag, and of course, my dog. We would take our dogs for a quick walk, unpack, freshen up, and then go to the most magical place in the world! No, not Disney world...Angelo's New York style pizza! There we would order a very large cheese pizza and either a glass of wine or a beer. Even though our combined body weight was less than 220 lbs., we would sit there until we finished the entire pizza, wine, and usually a few garlic rolls! Ah, the good old days and the joys of being unconscious.

But there is a point to my story. Years later I became vegan, and shortly after that, gluten free. Mary and I continued to visit each other, but my dietary changes left me with a choice of going to the health food store and buying an Amy's frozen, gluten-free, soy cheese pizza while Mary ordered take-out from Angelo's, OR keeping with our tradition for this one meal and dealing with the congestion, swollen eyes, and moderate constipation that was sure to arise the next day. My decision? You guessed it. Be proactive and take some herbs to ensure that things will clean out efficiently the day after our pizza party, and have fun with my cousin! It was a very, very conscious decision.

While some of you are balking at my "weakness," I can hear others cheering and chanting my name! The reality is that we will all fall to temptation at one time or another. But if we do this from a state of conscious awareness, it becomes easier to get back on track the next day. These days, since detox and eating raw, I make the choice to not have the pizza and I must say, I am still quite happy. The time spent with Mary far surpasses any pizza. Moreover, we have learned to create new rituals and traditions that feed our bodies and our souls.

Finally, I want to mention something about consciousness in relation to meditation. In the late 90's, I went to a three day workshop hosted by Deepak Chopra. It was an amazing time and I was in awe of this very famous man being so approachable. When asked a question by one of the participants regarding a personal challenge, Deepak would speak a bit on the topic, but at the end his answer would always be the same: "Meditate." This takes us full circle to the state of consciousness that we are working to achieve in our daily life choices.

Mediation is an extremely important component when incorporating consciousness into your life and your being. There are many, many forms of meditation, and I am here to tell you that I am no guru in this matter. But, what I can recommend, is that you try it. I am not suggesting that you convert from your current spiritual beliefs to a new one, nor am I trying to coax you into a religious or spiritual life. Meditation, and more specifically, *mindful meditation* is not a religion, it is a practice.

Mindful meditation is the simple and direct practice of moment-to-moment mindfulness. Through careful and sustained observation, the practitioner of mindful meditation experiences the ever-changing flow of the mind/body process. This awareness leads us to accept more fully the pleasure and pain, fear and joy, and sadness and happiness that life inevitably brings. Equanimity and peace develop as insight expands, bringing wisdom and compassion to ourselves and others. As we begin to practice mindful meditation, we become attuned to the understanding that conscious choices begin to happen more easily and with less struggle. I highly recommend that you check out our resource chapter to learn more about this.

Whatever form of mediation you currently practice or are interested in exploring more of, I encourage you to take the time to experience the change in your life through this simple repose.

"The greatest wealth is health."

- Virgil

C|U|R|E *quotes*

chapter eleven
"I can't afford to eat healthy food,"
and other impediments.

Day after day, my staff and I work with people from all over the world battling everything from weight issues to cancer. We serve them with love, compassion, and understanding, and ask just one thing in return: that they care as much about their own health as we do. That seems obvious and easy to do. After all, we are total strangers and could not possibly care about the health and well-being of our patients more than they care about themselves. Surprisingly though, it often seems that way. It seems that we are deeply connected to their success, sometimes more than they are. I have struggled to understand why that is. I have come to no clear conclusion, but what I have learned over the years is that there are legitimate and illegitimate excuses to participating in one's own healing process.

Let me first begin with illegitimate excuses, as there are no answers to these that would help a patient make the move to detoxification. It is the legitimate excuses that we can work through. An illegitimate excuse is the one that keeps changing. You know, when you ask your child why they didn't clean their room and the response changes by the second. "I didn't have enough time!" "I couldn't find the vacuum cleaner!" "I didn't hear you!" "My room is clean enough!" When one continues to come up with different reasons for the same question, you can be pretty sure that the excuse is not legitimate.

True legitimate excuses are the same each time you ask. When a legitimate excuse is met with a solution, the obstacle to detoxification is removed and the patient becomes eager to get started. So, what are some legitimate obstacles to detoxification, and more importantly, what are their solutions? Let's take a look.

I cannot afford to eat healthy food—this is one of the most common concerns of individuals interested in healing their body through detoxification. As many of you may know, fruits and vegetables (organic or conventionally grown) are far more expensive that they have ever been and certainly more expensive than pizza, a Big Mac, or even roasted chicken. The price per pound of some fruits or vegetables has quadrupled in the last decade while the cost of animal protein has shrunk in comparison. This is due greatly to government subsidies of the beef, pork, dairy and fowl industries.

Grains are also highly subsidized so that bread, cereal, and other processed grain products are put on the dining room table in every meal. In the meantime, produce subsidies are a fraction of their counterparts' making it near impossible for middle class families to purchase produce in any significant amount, and poor families rarely see a fresh piece of fruit or a salad on the table. I can go on and on about this issue which has no clear resolution to the systemic problem of food costs. For now, I will focus on solutions to the problem of day to day purchases of produce.

Please bear in mind that the solutions presented here are not for an all organic diet. Unfortunately, it is not always possible to find organic produce even if one can afford it. These solutions will help you to consume a complete fruit and vegetable diet during detox and allow you to keep a high amount of these lifesaving foods in your diet for years to come. Please also refer to the appendix for a list of the worst foods to eat, non-organic or conventionally grown.

The following are ideas for how to purchase more affordable produce. Not all solutions are available in your area. Be creative, become a detective and seek out live food!

> **Costco:** This is a well-known "warehouse" style store that has in recent years begun to carry more and more organic produce, both fresh and frozen. Their prices are tough to beat and the produce quality even rivals that of local grocery stores as well as "health food" stores like Whole Foods Market. Produce is usually seasonal which is also preferred. They also carry a nice variety of conventionally grown fruit and vegetables when organic is not available.

Sam's Club: Similar to Costco with less variety of organics, though they have improved more recently as well. Sam's Club is owned by the same family that started Walmart. I will take just a moment to address the fact that there has been much debate over this company as far as their employment practices and trade practices. Many people have chosen to boycott them and I completely understand if you choose to do so. However, I am not here to argue against them or on their behalf. My goal is to help you achieve your detox goals both physically and financially. It is your choice to decide how you feel about this company.

Walmart: Again, linked to Sam's Club. They too have increased organic produce, are in nearly every city and have significantly lower prices than local grocery stores and health food stores.

Farmer's markets: These are not always the best prices as some farmer's markets that pop up in larger cities just peddle grocery store produce that has been redistributed. However, many of them are true farmers' markets which support local farmers and can really provide reasonable prices with freshly picked produce. Ask them about bulk purchasing as this may glean an even better deal.

Food Co-ops: A co-operative (co-op) is an autonomous association of persons united voluntarily to meet their common economic, social, and cultural needs through a jointly-owned and democratic enterprise. In the case of food co-ops, their goal is to provide produce (often times organic) at a reasonable price on a weekly or biweekly basis. Usually you pay a set amount per month and you receive a box of produce. Some co-ops allow you to choose from a list of fruits and vegetables while others give you an equal share of whatever produce is purchased. Typically, it is locally grown and therefore only what is in season. Here is a national registry of co-ops:
http://www.coopdirectory.org/directory.htm

Online stores: In today's technologically driven world, you would be hard pressed to not find what you are looking for on the internet, even when it comes to food. While you can find online stores that sell fresh produce and deliver to your home, they may not always be cost effective. However, I have found that dried and dehydrated fruit and vegetables can be found much cheaper online. One of my favorite dried fruits are mulberries. At the local big chain health food store, eight ounces of these tasty morsels are a whopping $12.99! But online I have purchased 16 ounces of organic mulberries for $8.99!!! That is a savings of $16.99! Incredible! One of my favorite sites is **https://nuts.com/**.

Please see Chapter 14: "Recipes and resources" for an extended list of online stores.

Always ask: Throughout the course of my life I have found that if you do not ask, you will never know if something is possible. My motto (OK, one of my mottos) is *always ask.* Most of us go into our local grocery stores on a weekly basis. We get to know the cashiers, bag people and hopefully the manager. The grocery store staff tends to be quite friendly, helpful, and wants your business. If there is something I would like to purchase, but the store does not carry it, I will go to the manager and ask. There is a very good chance that they can order the product and are usually happy to do so. On another note, if you are in the process of detoxifying and are really loading up on fruit, vegetables for juicing, or even mono-fasting, this is the time to talk to the store manager or co-op organizer about bulk pricing. In many instances of detoxification, we ask our patients to dig deeper and go on some type of fast (see Chapter 8: "Steps to cure") like a grape-fast, for example. During a grape-fast, one can easily go through several pounds of grapes per day. Grapes, especially if they are organic, can be very pricey. But if you go to the store manager and inquire about purchasing a crate of grapes, pricing is often lower. This is true for all produce. Just foster a relationship with the store manager, co-op organizer, or vendor at the farmer's market and you can get great deals!

Time is on your side

Another obstacle to the detox process is time. In modern life we always seem to be on the go. Often both partners in a relationship work full time, and for the stay at home parents, there are carpools to school, dance classes, soccer practice, homework, and of course grocery shopping. By the time you get home from the tornado of life, who feels like prepping food? So what is the answer? Don't detox? Wait for a more convenient time? Hire a personal assistant? None of these responses are helpful or beneficial. The more reasonable answer is K.I.S.S. You know, Keep It Simply Silly. By that I mean eat like a monkey. Nibble, graze, munch, and snack. Fruit of course is the obvious choice. Grapes, bananas, berries, and apples are all very simple, easy, and convenient foods for snacking on the way to the office or PTA meeting. Many grocery stores now provide precut melon, mango, pineapple, or papaya packaged and ready to go. If you want to sip your breakfast, a smoothie can be easily thrown together by quickly peeling an orange or two and adding it to the blender with some frozen organic berries and precut pineapple. Make enough for 2–3 smoothies and you are good for three meals!

Adding vegetables to your detox could not be easier. Purchase a prewashed spring mix, spinach, or baby kale and follow your primate instincts by reaching in, grabbing a handful, and munching! Many grocery stores prepare mixed greens and veggie salad without dressing. Make your own and take it with you. Grab some baby bell peppers, celery, carrots, or cucumbers and dip them in guacamole or one of the dressings in this book. Bake several sweet potatoes at the beginning of the week and enjoy one every day with a fresh avocado. It's like butter, only better!

Don't forget, this is detox, not Martha Stewart! No need for fancy fooling around. Like the NIKE slogan says, *"Just do it!"* My job is to alkalize you, detoxify you, and set the stage for reversing disease and healing your body. I never said this would be a dance with the Galloping Gourmet! Simply put, don't let time stand in the way of healing. Your #1 priority is yourself!

Certainly, you will be amazed at how your taste buds begin to subtle differences between baby kale and baby spinach. Select the texture of cabbage over romaine lettuce for your veggie wrap and understand the necessity of juicing celery when you are craving salt. All in all, the detox process does not have to be complicated when it comes to your menu. Of course, if you have the time and the creativity, by all means go for it and invent new and exciting recipes. But if you don't have the time, keep it simple. Time is NOT a reason to deprive yourself of the greatest gift there is, the gift of regeneration. The gift of C.U.R.E.

"The only thing we have to fear is fear itself"

Emotions are another reason why people may choose to avoid detox. The emotion that I see most commonly is fear. Fear of eating fruit; fear of going hungry; fear of detox effects; fear of starting something new. Fear is a tremendous emotion that holds most of us back from achieving greatness, whether it be in our career, relationships, or health. I don't know how to help you overcome your fears. I just know that if you don't, you are destined to repeat your problems over and over and over again. Remember the definition of insanity: To keep doing what you have always done and expecting different results. The only way to see change in your body is to make changes in your habits. This is incredibly obvious and has been stated by people older, wiser, and greater than me. But truth is truth and it is time you face it. I have said it before and I will say it again and again. There is no greater, more holistic, or more profound way to reverse the process of disease and heal the body than this level of detoxification. Put fear aside and move forward...before it is too late.

Fear is also connected to our feelings regarding how we believe others perceive us. Everyone likes to be liked. We want to be part of the group and fit in. This is not limited to children or teenagers. Adults feel a strong sense of peer pressure as well, whether it be from friends, family, or co-workers. In our desire to fit in we can sabotage our health in the most dreadful way. Not being able to stand up for yourself in the face of the tribe (see Chapter 8) can lead you down a path of deteriorating health. When your parents asked "If Johnny jumped off the bridge, would you jump off too?" and you thought "What a stupid question! Of course I wouldn't," they were trying to prepare you for relationship challenges in the future. Little

Johnny is now John and he is handing you a beer and a rack of ribs and is taunting you about your man card being revoked if you turn down this hearty lunch for a wimpy salad! Maybe little Susie, now Susan, is questioning you as to why wine is not allowed on the detox. "It's only grapes" she says with a slur, "and besides, NBC's Dr. "S" says it is good to have a glass (or two) every day!"

Not for nothin', but I will start taking advice from the good doctor once they have reversed Grave's disease. Until then, leave detox to detox specialists and leave wine at the bar. Emotions, be it fear, insecurity, anger, anticipation, or worry can certainly derail us off the path of detox or even keep us from getting on in the first place. Don't let them. Create a new pattern, find a new tribe, go outside the box and trust yourself. If it is something that no one else is doing and insurance doesn't pay for, you are likely on the right track!

Vacations, holidays and other fun events
Holidays are wonderful times to gather with friends and family and celebrate religious occasions, commemorate a nation's history or ring in a new year. Unfortunately, holidays are also a very common excuse for why someone can't detox. *"Christmas is 3 weeks away. My birthday is coming up in two months. I am going away next summer."* In 14 years of practice, I have certainly heard it all. News flash—Christmas lasts 24 hours; 48 hours if you count Christmas Eve. The 4th of July is also 24 hours. The only people that can pull off an 8-day holiday excuse are my Jewish friends. And trust me, you can say no to latkes! OK, I know there are some important religious traditions that include certain foods that are not on the detox menu, but all of the days leading up to the holiday and even the hours leading up to the holiday meal can be spent eating fruits and vegetables. If you go off of your detox diet for that one holiday, wedding, or birthday meal it will not reverse the progress you would have made up to that point. But, if you wait for the perfect time to start detox when there are no holidays, vacations, or weddings to attend, then your next big event may just be your funeral. The truth is that there are lovely detox-friendly meals that I have brought to the holiday table during my year-long detox that my friends and family "just had to try!" leaving me to guard my food like a pit bull so that my husband and I would have enough. I have traveled on

cruises, to Disney World, and Canada with my mini blender in tow and a few specific directions to the wait staff at restaurants. This is not hard, just challenging. After all, aren't holidays and events about spending time with friends and family to celebrate the milestones of life? Have we gotten to the point in life where food is the party and people are secondary? If you are thinking about detoxifying your body, please do it. Do it now! The holidays will come and go. OK, eat some turkey, a slice of brisket, or some apple pie. But the next day, blend your smoothie, dig into a melon or make a mulberry "cereal" and feel the feeling of acid versus alkalinity.

My husband, wife, or other family member does not believe in detox

I realize that I was so truly blessed to have a husband who was not only supportive of the detoxification process, but who also wanted to experience it alongside me. Having his support made the process (nearly) effortless, especially when it came to shopping and preparing meals. I knew I would not have to prepare two different meals every night or defend why I was going through such a "strict" dietary process. Even though Anthony detoxed for 12 weeks compared to my 52 weeks, starting on the same page granted me an amazing start in the detox world. That being said, most individuals detox on their own. There are certainly those occasions where a friend, partner, or parent walks alongside someone who chooses the path of detox, but for the vast majority of people this is not the case. For those of you who go it alone, hurray for you! You have chosen the greatest gift that you could give yourself. But you still have to deal with family and friends. Remember, this is YOUR walk, not theirs.

I always encourage a new patient to bring in their significant other or someone they live with or spend a great deal of time with for the first visit. It is important for the other person to understand why we get sick, how the body works and the reasons for herbs and the dietary changes during detox, even though they are not necessarily joining the patient during the process. Teaching the how and why of detox to others will alleviate their desire to sabotage the process. For the vast majority of individuals that come to my office alone, I ask them to understand that they will be challenged by others and that knowledge is power. Take in as much information and knowledge as possible and then experience the benefits for yourself. Be the shining beacon for others to follow.

Ultimately, YOU have to be strong. YOU have to understand the process and make the choice that you are going to do this no matter what others might say. This is your body, your life, and your health. Never forget that. If you do, you will give up your opportunity to heal.

Where there is a will, there is a way

Lastly, I often field the question regarding willpower. This from women who have birthed children, individuals who performed surgery, litigated a murder trial, served in the military, built skyscrapers, taken care of sick parents, and put themselves through med school. Not to mention the firefighters and police officers who serve our community. It takes enormous strength and willpower to get through 10 years of school, put your life on the line for your fellow man, or squeeze a baby through a body part that is smaller than a dime! This is just detox, guys! Don't make that big of a deal out of the process! It is just a bunch of fruits and vegetables. There are currently millions of men, women, and children who are starving to death at this moment that would give their right arm and leg to eat even a fraction of the amazing bounty of food you will eat during detox. Stop! Stop your fear, stop your worrying, and yes, for a few days, tap into your reservoir of willpower. For it is only a few days that you will actually need willpower. After about 5–7 days, you will have the routine of detox down, and you will no longer feel hungry or get cravings, especially cravings of carbohydrates and sugar. If you consume enough calories for your energy requirements you will not be hungry. In those rare cases where hunger persists, it indicates an issue of adrenal fatigue and possible thyroid issues, which will then be supported with the appropriate herbs and gland tonic. The appropriate herbs will also work to cleanse the bowels so that absorption of nutrients can be improved. This will also help to curb hunger due to intestinal congestion leading to malabsorption.

The bottom line is excuses are like rear ends, everyone has one and they usually stink! So cross off your list of excuses and instead focus on what you can do. Heal your body from the inside out!

*"Rather than love, than money, than fame,
give me truth."*

- Henry David Thoreau

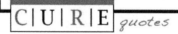 C | U | R | E quotes

chapter twelve
Testimonials

When I heard of Roseanne Calabrese' practice I was intrigued. It didn't matter that I was sent as a guinea pig (to check it out by my husband). All I knew was that the firefighters that went to see her looked 20 years younger, felt like never before, and had a reversal of serious health issues to being healthy again. All their aches and pains had vanished. I had to experience it for myself. Having battled high cholesterol for 10 years and nothing I did worked including never eating beef or pork, daily high aerobics and eating lean healthy, I decided to try it before submitting to Rx drugs.

The energy I felt once at Partners in Healing was remarkable. Everything I was hearing, I knew deep down inside was what I wanted: alternative medicine. I've read plenty on health and nutrition but didn't quite "get it". So I went all in with Rosanne and Diane. They were patient, extremely supportive, and marvelous! Every question was answered. It was my last try before beginning meds. I started with my detox at 269 total cholesterol on March 23, 2015. And just six weeks later I was at 238 and by September my total cholesterol was 218 without a single pill of what my doctor ordered! Just good old detoxification for 42 days and a plant based diet free of anything that has eyes, feet, and crawls! I gave up chicken and fish altogether! I lost 12 pounds and feel 21 at 45! My husband and children are eating 80% fruits for breakfast and more soups and salads as a result! Our lifestyle has changed for the better! My husband was sold and began his detox and lost 20 lbs., got his energy back and looks like he did when we first fell in love! Thank you Rosanne and your staff for giving us a new perspective on life: Live, love, and laugh on a healthy plant based living!

Emma Romero Rodriguez

Hi Roseanne,

I couldn't wait to email you. I know *Sarah* will be emailing you that she heard today that she no longer needs Methimazole! I am beyond thrilled! Her endocrinologist told her to keep doing whatever she is doing and to repeat bloodwork in a few weeks to be sure everything is going well.

She has worked so hard since she began in May. There have certainly been ups and downs. All that effort has paid off. I know she will continue to be in touch with you to see what else she can introduce and to be sure she maintains her health. We had a long talk over the weekend that so much of what she has learned and has done over the past months is now her new normal way of living.

I still can't believe how fortunate I was to find your site and connect with you. When you first talked with me, everything made sense, and that first conversation you had with *Sarah* made sense to her. Because you went through all of this yourself, she had faith that she could heal. Thank you so much for your wisdom, your guidance and your support. (Please thank Dee as well!)

With appreciation,

Caroline

I found Rosanne via an Internet blog while searching for an alternative solution to handling my recently diagnosed Graves' disease. The thought of losing my thyroid, as my body attacked it, made as much sense to me as arresting the customers in a bank during a bank robbery. She was extremely responsive and living proof that you can cure yourself of this "autoimmune" disease. She is kind, caring, supportive and the type of person all doctors should aim to emulate. It is because of Rosanne, I am now on a path to educate and help others.

Amy Richards

Where do I start in telling you the difference that Rosanne has made in my health and well-being...?

When I first met Rosanne I could not stand up more than 20 minutes before my lower back would start to hurt. The pain could get so severe that I had to sit down and rest until the pain would subside. Through the treatment from Partners in Healing, both acupuncture and massage therapy the pain is completely gone. I remember waking up after my daughter's wedding and saying to myself, "Wow!" I had absolutely no back pain whatsoever. I had none since and it's been over 7 years now.

Now let me say this about the cleanse and cell rejuvenation. I cannot believe the results. I am a Type 2 diabetic (for at least 20 years) and having a hard time keep it under control. Roseanne has said to me, "When you're ready to get rid of it let me know."

Well, after developing an infection on my leg, in which the doctor did not know what it was, I called Roseanne and said "I surrender, when can you see me?" We went over the plan and said I was to eat fruits and vegetables mostly, sweet or red potato. I reminded her that I am a diabetic and you want me to eat these fruits? Grapes, peaches, plums, watermelon etc. I haven't eaten them in 20 years. She said yes. To be honest I thought she was crazy and my sugar levels were going to go soooo high. But I know Roseanne, and with the trust that I have in her, I followed the plan.

The results so far (about five months): I have lost 40 pounds (10 more to go) My sugar levels are in control, in the morning 100 or less, was 200 before, evening the same, all while eating sweet fruit. My diabetic medicine is being reduced with my goal to eliminate them all. My MD doctor cannot believe it.

The best part is the compassion that Roseanne has. She does understand what you are going through and is always supporting you, never making you wrong when you have slips etc.

I am so glad that we have found each other.

David Blumstein

In August 2012 I had just graduated from college and almost simultaneously reached one of the most desperate points in my life. Four years prior, I was involved in a car accident in which I sustained a severely shattered pelvis. After many months recovering, I thought I had returned to my normal life only to have my first attack. My stomach could not keep any food in it, whatsoever. For the next four years, my diet would get more and more narrow until most days I was only having little bits of broth and rice. As a result I began having other issues with sleep and energy—I would sleep for days and wake up tired, my skin was breaking out for the first time in my life, my lymph nodes in my neck and underarms were swollen to the size of small eggs, and my stress was absolutely through the roof.

I pushed myself through four years of college like this, never addressing the issue until immediately after graduation when I couldn't look away anymore. My stomach issues had gotten so bad that I had not been able to keep any bit of food in my body for two full weeks. I was malnourished and I felt myself fading. I thought, I'm not eating, how long can this go on before I die?

That was when I came to Rosanne. I sat down with her for a consultation, for the first time admitting everything I had been suffering with for so many years. She heard my desperation, let me cry, and then began to explain about the three main components of the body (blood, cells, and lymph, anyone?). She broke down her plan into easily digestible parts, no pun intended. She let me choose how fast I would transition to an anti-inflammatory diet. We worked up from very small amounts of herbal liquids to small amounts of herbal capsules. And most of all, she was there in full support of me, as was her staff; be it a phone call, an emergency appointment, I felt I had the support I needed to take on the task of healing myself.

The day after seeing Rosanne, I took my first bite of food in weeks, a small amount of watermelon, and did not get sick (it is still my favorite food). I had been so toxic from my experience in the hospital after my car accident (think IV painkillers, antibiotics, radiation) compounded with the stress of recovery and lasting PTSD, my body had become completely and chronically inflamed.

The alkaline food Rosanne recommended actually worked with my system, when nothing else did. For the next 16 weeks, I dove into the plan we created and I watched my body morph. I did not have any of the same issues I had been having, although I did experience detox symptoms, all of which were professionally and compassionately managed by the crew at Partners In Healing. I derived motivation from the changes I was seeing and my appointments with Rosanne. And I even watched lifelong issues with energy, ADD, and depression melt away. I felt better than I ever had and I was working for it! It was amazing to have control over my body and my health again. I was able to return to normal activities, search for a job, see my friends and family, instead of constantly feeling incapacitated and trapped.

My experience with Rosanne and the C.U.R.E. program gave my life back to me; something I thought might never happen after that fateful day I was involved in the crash. I have since integrated all I've learned from my time healing myself to manage my PTSD and inflammatory conditions. I know how to stave it off completely; I know how to let it ebb and flow as life happens. And most importantly, I know how to take control and prevent disease from taking over my life again.

Shortly after my own detoxification period, I began working with Rosanne's patients helping them navigate the food aspect of detoxification. I shared my recipes that satisfied my cravings and I taught them techniques I learned that made this lifestyle a live-able reality. That is how much I believe in the change the C.U.R.E. program can create in you. Inflammation is so often at the root of our ailments, and giving your body real food and fuel for the amazing mechanisms it is trying to perform is step one in healing yourself and allowing yourself to get better. I have since opened up a vegan, gluten-free restaurant with these principles in mind, with a detoxification-friendly menu planned, and with the ability to cater to those who are healing themselves through food. It is another aspect of support that has stemmed from Partners in Healing and I am very proud to be able to contribute to all those who may take the same journey that I did four years ago.

Experiencing the C.U.R.E. program empowered me and gave me the tools to heal myself through natural means when medical means could not help me and doctors had no answers for me. It left me endowed with information and empowerment that I could not ignore when moving forward in my life and set me up on a path I would have never imagined: one of owning a restaurant and working with food every day, coming up with ways to make healthy food delicious and comforting. Taking a chance on a new way of life, may bring you so much more than health (although simply healing would be a beautiful and worthy reason on its own), it may bring you a purpose you had never recognized, or an understanding of yourself you did not previously possess, and for that I am forever grateful.

Sincerely,

Ann Nacknouck

Owner of Clovermint of Café & Market

Nutritional detox, under the guidance of Dr. Calabrese, not only saved my life but gave me a quality of life I had never known. After being diagnosed with an autoimmune disease at age 7, I spent my entire life being sick with one ailment or another such as chronic sinus infections, IBS, and sore throats. In my late 30's, my immune system stopped working properly after my NK (a/k/a Killer Cells) stopped functioning. This allowed my body to contract and re-activate no less than 9 different viruses - simultaneously. I was subsequently diagnosed with Chronic Fatigue Immune Dysfunction Syndrome, Fibromyalgia, Chronic Epstein-Barr, and several other ailments. Then my body kicked in an auto-immune response to fight the viruses and started attacking itself. I saw every kind of medical specialist and took numerous medications, including a pill form of chemotherapy. Since Western medicine was not solving the problems, I decided to try a different route and made an appointment with Dr. Calabrese. She guided me through nutritional detox and how to maintain a healthy plant-based diet. She utilized herbs and acupuncture and within two months, I started feeling better than I had since I was a kid. A year and a half-later I am happy to report that I am healthier than I have ever been. I am living proof that eating a plant-based diet can save your life.

Wendy G.

I've been working with Rosanne for over three years now and I have seen numerous results while detoxing. The most important one is that I am 35 years old and for most of my life I've had very painful menstrual cycles, and sometimes I would skip months at a time, for numerous years. Since I've been seeing Rosanne I have not skipped one menstrual cycle and my menstrual cycles are painless, much shorter and less intense. I have removed significant toxins from my body. I used to suffer from numerous pain, ailments and discomforts like plantar fasciitis, back pain, sciatica and neck pain due to herniated and/or bulging disks. I don't suffer from that anymore. I used to have headaches and migraines, almost on a weekly basis. Since detoxing with Rosanne, I can not remember the last time I had a migraine. Headaches in general are very very rare now, if I do get one it's usually due to toxic smells in my environment. When I'm active in the detox, I sleep better as my sleeping cycle regulates. I am a night owl and have shift work, so my sleep schedule is usually out of whack. However, when detoxing my sleep cycle is that of a person that works a normal 9 to 5 type job. I'm ready for bed by 10 PM and I'm awake by 7 AM, and I have a lot more energy. Once I completed the detox cycles my cholesterol had dropped significantly by 20 points and my triglycerides dropped about 30 points. I've removed about 35 pounds from my frame. In addition to the detox, Rosanne has treated me with acupuncture, which has helped tremendously with the body pains. I've have also had treatments with the other practitioners in her office such as lymphatic massages and craniosacral massages. I am genetically predisposed for arthritis and bone degeneration diseases as well as heart disease. Rosanne is helping me reverse those genes so that I can live a long pain-free life. Rosanne is also helping me remove more weight from my frame so that I can soon bear kids. The most amazing part of the whole experience is that in addition to her knowledge, Rosanne is a truly unique person. When you're working with her, she not only gives you her knowledge, the herbs, and the practitioners, but she puts her heart into your treatment. She pours in her dedication. We live in a world where the doctors either want to cut you open and remove parts of your body or they want to give you some kind of medicine or chemicals to temporarily resolve your issue and make money. Rosanne gives you her dedication, she gives you her knowledge, and she gives herself whole heartedly, and what a trifecta that is!! I truly believe that with Rosanne on your side, any disease or issue you may have CAN be reversed! She truly is an angel!!! I am blessed to also call her my friend!

Zulge Guerra

Hi guys, in case you are wondering what I have been doing.. for the last 2 months I have followed a detox protocol. Fruits all day and vegetables (raw or cooked at night). I have also taken detox herbs. I have Grave disease, like my brother and my mother. The awesome news is that looks like I am doing really well. I just found out I will be on the lowest dose of medication for a while. hopefully, I can heal entirely soon. No one believes me, but I believe in the power of fruits and vegetables. I have been doing the detox with Rosanne Calabrese. I was diagnosed with Graves 2 and a half months ago and I did not lose any time and did extensive research on the internet and fell over Rosanne's blog. She also healed with Dr Morse protocol. I am also taking meds, I started with 30 mg of Methimazole per day and beta blockers. but honestly if you ask me, I think it is this protocol that is helping me heal. Mow, just 2 months later, I will be on 5 mg Methimazole and no beta blockers. that is an amazing improvement considering 90% of people with grave's disease get radiated and have their thyroid destroyed.

Happy healing to everyone!

M.P.

"Start by doing what's necessary;
then do what's possible;
and suddenly you are doing the impossible."

- Francis of Assisi

C | U | R | E *quotes*

"Invasive plants—Earth's way of insisting we notice her medicines."

- Stephen Harrod Buhner

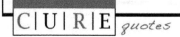

chapter 13
Appendix: Herbs; Clean food; Fasting; Acid/alkaline scale and list; Iridology chart

Exploring the power of herbal therapy

Herbology (the use of herbs for supporting, nourishing, and healing the body) basically began when man took his first breath. Not only were all of the fruits of the trees gifts from God for us to nourish the body, but plants known as herbs—their bark, stems, leaves, and roots—were gifts to ward off infection, kill unfriendly parasites, clean, heal, and rejuvenate our cells. There are countless herbs with healing properties on this planet, while hundreds, if not thousands still remain undiscovered. Every native culture in every region of the globe has its own indigenous healing herbs that are transformed into powerful teas, tinctures, powders, salves, and tablets.

In the course of my education to become a practitioner of traditional Chinese medicine (Eastern medicine), I learned that herbs were of the utmost importance when it came to bringing balance to the body. In TCM, herbs were rarely used as single remedies. Instead, ancient Chinese practitioners figured out ways to mix or blend herbs so that their properties would balance each other out, never allowing an herb to be too strong, harsh, cooling, warming, or purging. The art of creating formulas is indeed a gift requiring much study, as well as many hours of clinical experience. The authorities of traditional Chinese herbal therapy used their own bodies as their laboratories, testing herbal formulas on themselves before venturing out into a clinical setting.

At my clinic, Partners in Healing, I utilize both Eastern and Western herbs. I am blessed to have had an incredibly knowledgeable herbal instructor, Fu Di, at ATOM (Atlantic Institute of Oriental Medicine). is expertise in mixing Chinese herbal formulas was invaluable to my practice and methodology. Later in my career, as a result of my personal battle with Grave's disease, I was equally as fortunate to meet my mentor doctor Robert Morse. In my opinion, he is one of the foremost authorities on Western herbs and herbal formulations. All that I know regarding Western herbal formulas, I am proud to say, I have learned from him. As a practitioner, I have discovered the art of prescribing formulas based on correlations between an individual's medical history, iridology analysis, and physical constitution.

While Eastern and Western herbs are certainly not known to have dangerous or serious side effects such as those common to prescription and over the counter drugs, there are times when certain herbs are absolutely contraindicated for particular conditions, so I feel it is important to have a clinical and working knowledge of herbs in order to minimize uncomfortable effects and maximize healing. Working with a knowledgeable practitioner is paramount to gaining an optimal healing response. Therefore, I am going to touch on some basic herbs and their properties in this section, but I advise you to seek out the help of a detox specialist whether it be me or one of my many colleagues across the world, to guide you more specifically and individually.

I also encourage you to look into different herbal books regarding Naturopathy, TCM, Ayuverda and other native cultures.

Properties of Chinese herbs

According to TCM, each herb has a specific action or actions. This holds true in Western herbology as well, although the properties may be utilized in different ways. In TCM the actions of herbs are listed below.

1. **Harmonizing**: Herbs used to regulate the physiological functions; achieve balance of organs (spleen and liver) as well as digestive issues.

2. **Purgative**: Herbs which break down the internal accumulations via the bowels. In TCM, while purgative herbs are used as laxatives for relieving intestinal stagnancy, they

also function in the removal of heat, fire, toxins and retained fluids. Individuals usually present with fullness, distention and pain in the gastric and abdominal regions, constipation, and poor appetite.

3. **Heat clearing**: These herbs treat various heat syndromes through the actions of clearing away heat, draining fire, cooling blood, and eliminating the associated toxicity while nourishing the body. Classic heat signs include high fever, profuse sweating, a surging pulse, excessive thirst, bleeding, and altered consciousness as well as ulcerated skin sores.

4. **Warming**: These herbs warm the interior and unblock meridians to eliminate "cold" conditions inside the body. This is known as restoring yang-qi. Conditions include chills, fatigue, gastric discomfort, increased urine output, and loose bowels.

5. **Tonic or tonifying**: Herbs in this category enrich, augment, nourish or replenish the qi, blood, yin and yang. This will cover a multitude of deficiency ailments.

6. **Astringent**: These herbs arrest abnormal discharge or leakage of fluids and other substances from the body, such as sweat, sputum, blood, urine, stool, sperm, and vaginal discharges and are almost always used with tonifying herbs.

7. **Calming**: Herbs in this category relieve mental tension and uneasiness and are similar to anxiety medications of the West.

8. **Orifice opening**: Herbs used in cases of loss of consciousness, delirium, epilepsy and convulsions. These herbs tend to be quite aromatic.

9. **Qi regulating**: Herbs that regulate the flow of qi (vital energy) through organs and meridians.

10. **Blood regulating**: Herbs which treat disorders related to blood flow (blood in TCM is known as fluid inside the blood

vessels that provides nutrition and lubrication for the body), from relieving blood stasis to arresting bleeding.

11. **Dampness dispelling**: Herbs which address sluggishness, tiredness, heavy limbs, a feeling of distention in the head, stiffness and pain in the joints, or limb puffiness; bodily discharges will tend to be sticky and turbid.

12. **Phlegm resolving**: Herbs in this category address what TCM calls disharmony of body fluids which can produce either external visible phlegm, (i.e. sputum secreted by the respiratory tract) or internal invisible phlegm due to dysfunction of the lungs and the spleen, and sometimes by the consumption of body fluids by fire and heat evils. Formation of phlegm is responsible for the occurrence and development of a range of disorders, such as coughing, wheezing, nausea, dizziness or vertigo, nodules or lumps, and seizures.

13. **Wind eliminating**: Herbs which address both external (body surface, muscles, bones, tendons, joints and meridians and thus lead to headache, itching, skin rash, numbness, spasms, and movement difficulty in the joints as in colds, flu etc.) and internal (characterized by dizziness, vertigo, tremors, convulsions, loss of muscle tone, difficulty in speaking, sudden loss of consciousness, facial distortion and paralysis as in a stroke) wind disorders.

14. **Dryness moisturizing or yin nourishing**: Herbs that address both external and internal sources which consume body fluid and causes fluid loss. Symptoms may include dry, wrinkled, or withered skin, dry hair and scalp, dry mouth and cracked lips, dry and hard stools or headache, cough, throat soreness and secretions, thirst and pant.

15. **Exterior relieving**: Herbs which relieve "exterior syndrome" with emerging symptoms of chills, fever, headache, and generalized aching.

16. **Digestive supporting**: These herbs address a broad spectrum of digestive issues including distention and fullness in the gastric and abdominal regions, poor appetite, bad breath, belching, nausea, thick and greasy tongue coat, loose bowels and sometimes diarrhea.

In Western herbology, the herbs are classified as such:

1. **Adaptogens**: A diverse group of herbs that aid in handling the body's stress responses. These herbs restore overall balance and strengthen the functioning of the body as a whole without impacting the balance of an individual organ or body system. They can be stimulating and/or relaxing, and can improve focus, support immune system functionality, balance blood pressure, or any number of other physiological imbalances. Examples of adaptogens include: Garlic, Echinacea, gingko, goldenseal, licorice, basil, and rhodiola.

2. **Anhydrotics**: These herbs assist in stopping excess sweating (e.g. Agrimony, Buchu, Butcher's Broom).

3. **Astringents**: Herbs with drying, drawing, and constricting effects to help create a barrier for healing. Look for that "puckered" feeling as in eating a lemon. They can be used topically to ease bug bites and burns, help pull out splinters or infection from a wound, dry out oozing sores, tighten tissue and gums, tone the skin, and stop bleeding. Astringent herbs also work internally to help tone mucus membranes and dry up conditions of excess, like diarrhea, too much urine, or profuse sweating. (These include Agrimony, Bugleweed, Horsetail, White Oak Bark, and Witch Hazel.)

4. **Alteratives**: Herbs that support your body's own natural defenses in the presence of illness and help restore proper function. Also known as "blood cleansers;" this action can occur through the lymph, glands, or mucus membranes. (Commonly used alteratives include Echinacea, Goldenseal, Sanicle, Yellow Dock)

5. **Anthelmintics**: Herbs capable of destroying or eliminating parasitic worms, especially human intestinal helminths (e.g. Bistort, Wormwood, Black Walnut).

6. **Anti-arthritics**: Reduce and reverse joint pain, swelling and stiffness including gout (e.g. Black Cohosh, Chaparral, Dandelion, Yellow Dock).

7. **Antifungals**: Destroy or prevent the growth of fungal infections (e.g. Wormwood, black walnut hull, Pau d'Arco Bark).

8. **Antibacterials**: Herbs that kill or reduce populations of harmful bacteria without destroying beneficial bacteria (e.g. black walnut, worm seed, cat's claw, fennel).

9. **Anti-inflammatory**: Herbs that counteract or diminish inflammation in addition to exhibiting vascular constrictive properties (e.g. yucca, devil's claw, wild yam, turmeric).

10. **Antiseptics**: These herbs help prevent the growth of microbes and cripple their activity. They can also aid in preventing or dealing with sepsis. A few examples of Western antiseptic herbs include Buchu, Burdock Leaves, Chamomile, Cayenne, and Echinacea.

11. **Aphrodisiacs**: Herbs that help stimulate sexual arousal through varied actions including increased circulation, relaxation, stimulation, or tonics that strengthen glandular health (e.g. Damiana, False Unicorn, Saw Palmetto, Yohimbe).

12. **Aromatics**: Herbs containing essential oils that present strong aromas. Most often used to stimulate the digestive system, reproductive system, and disinfect the respiratory tract, or help expectorate the lungs. Some aromatics are also excreted through the urinary tract or the skin. Common aromatics include Anise, Fennel, and Peppermint.

13. **Bitter tonic, bitters**: Herbs that help stimulate appetite and digestion by getting gastric juices flowing and your

peristalsis moving. Small amounts (1–2 drops) on the tongue may be all that is required to activate the production of beneficial digestive secretions including saliva, gastric acid, and bile. Helpful for constipation, gas related cramping, sluggish digestive movement, and to support a healthy appetite after an illness (e.g. Gentian, Chaparral, Wormwood).

14. **Calming Nervines**: These herbs specifically support the nervous system, so not all calming herbs are nervines. Calming herbs have a range of actions including tonic nervines, mildly calming, anti-spasmodic, and strongly sedative. They are used to relieve nagging muscle tension and spasms, some kinds of pain, circular thoughts, insomnia, and occasional worry (e.g. Skullcap, catnip chamomile, valerian).

15. **Carminitives**: These herbs are often aromatic and help expel gas from the digestive system. This action can help ease bloating and gas related cramping (e.g. fennel, caraway, peppermint).

16. **Cathartics**: Herbs that are active purgatives to the intestinal tract, exciting peristalsis and stimulating glandular secretions, producing semi-fluid bowel movements with some irritation and griping. They are also serve as powerful healers of the GI tract (e.g. Black, Hellebore, Culvers Root, Senna Leaves).

17. **Cell proliferants**: These herbs promote rapid healing and regeneration of the cells. (Aloe Vera, Comfrey, Elecampane, Saw Palmetto).

18. **Cholagogues**: These herbs have the specific effect of **stimulating the flow of bile from the liver into the intestines** (e.g. Beets, Fringetree, Mandrake).

19. **Demulcents**: Herbs that are mucilaginous and produce slime that coats, soothes, and protects mucus membranes triggering a reflex that helps promote natural moistening secretions

within the body systems such as respiratory, digestive, renal, and reproductive (e.g. slippery elm, comfrey, licorice).

20. **Depuratives**: Herbs that are considered to have purifying and detoxifying effects. Herbs that are considered depuratives include Blessed Thistle, Blue Flag, and Dandelion.

21. **Diaphoretics**: These herbs help raise your body temperature to make you sweat and stimulate circulation and increased perspiration. Using diaphoretics may be helpful for breaking dry fevers, erupting skin infections, promoting blood flow to cold extremities, and detoxification (e.g. Centaury, Coltsfoot, Sassafras).

22. **Diuretic**: Herbs that make you urinate. They help promote the elimination of fluids by increasing the amount of urine expelled by the kidneys. This can be helpful for water retention and urinary tract flushing (e.g. Tansy, Uva Ursi, Stone Root, Dandelion).

23. **Emmenagogues**: Herbs and remedies that stimulate and regulate menstrual flow and function. In most herbal texts the term is used in the wide sense of a remedy that normalizes and tones the female reproductive system (e.g. Saw Palmetto, False Unicorn, Nettle).

24. **Emollients**: These herbs are used as topical applications to help soothe, condition, and protect the skin (aloe vera, comfrey, marshmellow, plantain).

25. **Expectorants**: Herbs that encourage productive coughing by breaking up mucus in the lungs and expelling it more effectively (e.g. ececampane, mullein, and horehound).

26. **Laxatives**: herbs that in some way stimulate the bowels to promote bowel movements.

   - **Stimulating Laxatives:** Senna, turkey rhubarb, cascara, burdock, and yellow dock
   - **Bulking laxatives**: Flax, psyllium, and marshmellow

27. **Nutritives**: Herbs which nourish the body and supply material for tissue rebuilding (e.g. nettle, wild oats, horsetail, red clover, red raspberry leaf, chamomile, and alfalfa leaf).

28. **Purgatives**: Herbs that promote the vigorous evacuation of the bowels; usually used to relieve severe constipation (e.g. cascara, senna, fennel).

29. **Stimulants**: Increase functional activity and energy in the body, strengthening metabolism and circulation (e.g. Feverfew, Ginseng, Prickly Ash, Red Clover, rosemary, Wormwood, Yarrow).

30. **Stomachics**: Strengthen the functions of the stomach and help promote digestion, appetite, and relieve indigestion (e.g. Slippery Elm Bark, Gentian Root, Wild Yam Root).

31. **Tonics**: Herbs that stimulate nutrition and increase systemic tone, energy, and vigor. Enhances the entire system (e.g. Angelica, Centaury, Boneset, German Chamomile, Red Clover, Sanicle, Self-Heal, Stinging Nettle, Yarrow).

32. **Vermifuges**: Herbs which cause the expulsion or repulsion of intestinal worms and tapeworms (e.g. burdock root, wormwood, black walnut).

33. **Vulneraries**: Assist in healing of wounds by protecting against infection and stimulating cell growth (e.g. Agrimony, Balm of Gilead, Bladderwrack, Cleavers, Comfrey, Elder, Rue).

Clean food: The dirty dozen and then some

According to the EWG—the Environmental Working Group (a non-profit, non-partisan organization dedicated to protecting human health and the environment; www.EWG.org) you have a right to know about the safety of your environment including how toxic your food is. Here are some of the categories of foods that you should be informed of. Please keep in mind that the lists of food in each category change each year as new information is available.

The dirty dozen: Conventionally grown produce for 2016 with the highest pesticide load:
Apples, peaches, nectarines, strawberries, grapes, celery, spinach, sweet bell peppers, cucumbers, cherry tomatoes, imported snap peas and potatoes. In previous years, strawberries, sweet potatoes and other berries were high on the list. This does not mean that these foods are no longer toxic, just that they are not in the top 12. I caution you to look at previous lists and make your choices from a broader perspective. Use their website as a guide.

EWG's Clean Fifteen™ list of produce least likely to hold pesticide residues consists of avocados, sweet corn, pineapples, cabbage, frozen sweet peas, onions, asparagus, mangoes, papayas, kiwis, eggplant, grapefruit, cantaloupe, cauliflower and sweet potatoes. Relatively few pesticides were detected on these foods, and tests found low total concentrations of pesticides on them.

Fasting efficiently and safely

Today, fasting is used for things like rapid weight loss or to "kick-start" a diet. In naturopathy, fasting was an integral part of healing the body. There are so many fascinating books about fasting, from Upton Sinclair's *The Fasting Cure,* published in 1911, to Dr. Joel Furman's *Fasting and Eating for Health* published in 1995. Fasting has been a part of man's journey since the dawn of time. Whether it was done for spiritual reasons (found in all religious texts and spiritual practices), health benefits, or political/social statements (Gandhi), fasting has moved us through difficult times to bring us to a brighter future. When applying fasting to our place as part of the natural world, we understand that even animals utilize the power of fasting.

The choice to fast is driven by the necessity to heal. To bring rest to the digestive process and instead direct the body's energies elsewhere. During detoxification, eating only fruits and vegetables can be considered a "fast" for most people. But this form of detoxification does not allow for complete bowel rest and sometimes the body can reach a plateau when the digestive system still has to work, stagnating the cleansing and healing process. The body's ability to auto-lyse (break down non-essential tissue such as tumors or cysts) is sped up when other systems of the body are able to rest. That is where stricter fasting comes in.

There are actually several types of fasting. As stated earlier, consuming only fruits and vegetables can be considered a fast. Eating a single food, like grapes for instance, is called mono-fasting. There is also water fasting, lemon-water fasting, and dry fasting. I personally have never dry-fasted and therefore feel that I hold no authority to speak about it or recommend it. I also feel that both dry fasting and water fasting should be supervised by a physician or other authority and again I do not recommend it in the context of this book. In this section however, I will talk about two forms of fasting that are safe to do in short stints. Anywhere from 2 to 10 days can be easily tolerated provided:

- That at least 4 weeks of a clean, detox diet is done first.

- That the last 2-3 days before a fast is spent on fruit ONLY.

- That you are not in a weakened state.

- That you listen to your body and stop the fast if healing crises become too strong or you feel that the fast has weakened you too much.

- That you come off of the fast correctly and at the appropriate time.

Please know that everyone is different regarding fasting. For some, by the end of day one, there may be no feelings of hunger whatsoever. For me, it took until the morning of day two. I was certain going to bed that first night that I was going to wake up ravenous and abandon my fast. To my surprise I awoke feeling quite content so I soldiered on, deciding to take it day by day. For others, hunger may linger for two or three days. Persevere. The feeling of lightness and detachment from those urges is just around the bend.

I would like you to consider 10 days of whichever fast you choose. But be conscious! Listen to your body. Interpret its signs and signals. Understand healing crises and what to expect during your fast. The list of healing crises in Chapter 8: "Steps to C.U.R.E.," are possible during detoxification *and* during fasting. If at any time you do not feel strong enough to continue, by all means stop. However, you must follow the instructions discussed in the section below, **Breaking your fast**.

When deciding the best time to fast, I believe that less is more. Pick a time when you don't have a lot going on in terms of work, social life, family obligations etc. Few of us have the ability to just stay home and do nothing and for most people, there is no need to bring activity down to that level. You can continue about your regular routine with a few small changes. Do not exercise; rest when you feel the need; manage stress with mediation, prayer, or breath work.

Lastly, please stay hydrated. There are no dry-fasts in this book. You will either grape fast or lemon fast. Both include a good bit of liquid. If you find yourself getting thirsty, drink more lemonade, grape juice or consume more grapes. Do not become dehydrated.

Herbs and medications while fasting

Unless you are being supervised by a practitioner, I advise you *not* to discontinue any of your prescription medication. Keep in mind that with several weeks of a fruit and vegetable detox, and now fasting, there is a very good chance that you will need less of your blood pressure, diabetes, or thyroid medication—just to name a few. Monitor your vital signs (blood pressure, pulse, temperature, blood sugar etc.) and request a blood test to determine if meds should be reduced. It is always recommended that you communicate these findings with your doctor so that they can decide on updated medication dosages.

I have seen many of my patients' high blood pressure, high sugar, or hyperthyroid conditions rapidly stabilize after just a few weeks of detox. Monitor your numbers and *how you feel* so that you can make intelligent and informed decisions.

Generally speaking, herbs can be continued, though dosages may need to be reduced as there is no food present to buffer absorption. The act of fasting speeds up detox as well as healing so herbs may actually be more potent. Here comes that word again…be *conscious*! I am entrusting you with a lot. Mindfulness and attention to your body is fundamental.

Many versions of these fasts exist, some including things like enemas or "salt water flushes." They can be harsh, cause dehydration, or even a purging effect. I prefer to take a gentler approach. Some individuals experience a "backed-up" feeling when they start a fast. This is unpleasant but can hinder the body's ability to remove waste leading to a strong sense of ill feeling. Therefore, I recommend that you use either an herbal tea or capsule to be certain that bowels are moving. At least one bowel movement a day is expected while fasting, though three or more could occur in the beginning. Toward the end of the fast you may average less than one per day.

Breaking your fast
Breaking a fast is as crucial as starting one, if not more so. Knowing how and when to break a fast will determine the effectiveness of the fast. Trying to fast for too long or breaking the fast because of cravings will not propagate forward strides in healing. Understanding the difference between hunger and cravings is essential in determining when to end a fast.

Most of us do not know true hunger. We eat so much and so often that we do not give our brain time to catch up with our body. We also feel that an "emptiness" in the stomach is an indication of hunger. It is not. When fasting there is no doubt that the stomach is essentially empty. Yet the feeling of hunger does not arise. It is understanding your body and tapping into its energy that allows you to persevere without issue. Once hunger does creep up you will know its distinctive feeling. It will not take you by surprise, but allow you the time to make the decision to break-fast.

Outside of hunger, there are other reasons to break a fast. For example, if you have a difficult time balancing your blood sugar whether it be too high or too low, you may need to ease off of the fast. Hypo-glycemia (low blood sugar) tends to be more common than hyper-glycemia. Certainly it is expected that those numbers will possibly become unstable at times during your fast. But if you just cannot seem to level them out, it is time to ease back into food. Return to your fruit and vegetable detox and attempt another fast in a month or two. If symptoms listed in *cleansing effects and healing crises* persist for more than two days at a high level, or you just feel too uncomfortable to continue, you may also ease back into food, but **follow these instructions**:

For every three days of fasting you undergo, you should have 1–2 days of fresh fruit juice. I prefer orange juice but you can juice just about any fruit.

- **Day 1–2** – Orange Juice – up to 3 1-liter jars of fresh squeezed orange juice

- **Day 3** – Whole Fruit and Vegetable Juice

- **Day 4** – Raw Fruits and Vegetable

- **Day 5** – Regular Diet; detox or post detox diet.

Grape or grape juice fasting

Grape juice fasting uses much less digestive energy than grapes eaten in their whole form. But for those who wish to go longer than 10 days, grapes in their whole state can be more sustainable. If you are eating whole grapes be sure to have enough on hand to support your caloric and hydration needs. Also know that you may desire water while fasting on whole grapes. If so, drink mineral or spring water.

Organic grapes are always best, and those grown conventionally in the United States are next. For detox purposes, stay away from grapes grown outside of the US (unless you live in Europe or other Eastern nations).

Grape Juice

A juice extractor or juicer is necessary (please see resources chapter).
Juice a quart of grapes (seeds and small stems as well).
Any type of grape is acceptable, however the dark, seeded grapes are the best for fasting and detoxing in general.

There is no serving size during detox or fasting. You may drink grape juice as much and as often as you like. Grapes are high in antioxidant and astringent properties, which will aid in pulling toxins from the body.

Lemonade fast
This fast has been around in one form or another for many years. It has been used by naturopaths and natural hygienists for bowel rest, detoxing, and healing. The astringent value of lemons is amazing! Just think about a lemon's ability to get you to salivate just from cutting into it! This is nature's way of purging and "pulling" waste and toxins.

Directions:

2 tbsp. of fresh lemon or lime juice (approx. 1/2 lemon) – Never use pre-squeezed juice in those little plastic containers.

1/2 to 3/4 tbsp. genuine pure maple syrup (not maple-flavored sugar syrup) – the darker the better.

Pinch of Cayenne pepper (optional) as it also increases warmth and can add an additional lift. For those not used or averse to hot peppers, start with a dash and increase it as you are able.

Combine the juice, maple syrup, and cayenne pepper in a 10-ounce glass Mason jar or glass water bottle and fill with tepid or hot distilled or reverse osmosis water. (Cold water may be used if preferred.) Depending on what part of the world you are in, the temperature of the water can help keep you warm or cool you off.

Pure sorghum, black strap molasses, or coconut nectar (ask your local health food store or search on line) may be used as a lesser replacement when maple syrup is not available or if you do not like it.

For ease of fast, if you are traveling or working you can make a quart at a time.
10 cups distilled water
1 1/2 cup of fresh lemon juice
1/2 cup of pure maple syrup or the like

Shake well and refrigerate.

No other food or drink is taken outside of herbal tea for bowels and lemonade. You may consume as much and as often as you want. The key is to not allow hunger to creep in, so keep sipping!

Understanding specific foods and their acid/alkaline levels
There are various lists on the internet and in books that categorize and rate the level of acid and alkalizing responses in the human body to specific foods. This list is just one of them. While most resources agree about the majority of foods' acid and alkaline impact on the body, as you would expect, there are some discrepancies. Try not to get too bogged down by these small details. Just use this list as a guide, especially for post detox.

Also, it is important to keep in mind that just because a food falls in the category of "alkaline," does not mean it is allowed during detoxification. There are certain alkaline foods like hemp seeds or millet which are too high in protein during detoxification. High protein stresses the kidneys and therefore is not advised during this time.

Guidelines for determining acid/alkaline levels of foods
- For any food that has been cooked, frozen or canned, subtract 0.5 (raw juices, chemical-free dried foods are excluded).

- For any foods gown with chemicals, processed with chemicals, or prepared with sugar subtract 1.0

- The fresher and sweeter the food tastes, the higher its alkalinity.

Acid/Alkaline Scale

	7.5	
Extremely	7	Alkaline
	6.5	
Moderately	6	Alkaline
	5.5	
Slightly	5	Alkaline
	4.5	
Neutral	4	Neutral
	3.5	
Slightly	3	Acidic
	2.5	
Moderately	2	Acidic
	1.5	
Extremely	1	Acidic
	0.5	

FRUITS

ALKALINE-FORMING FOODS

Apples	5.5–6.0
Apricots	6.0
Avocados	6.0
Bananas	6.0
Berries	6.0
Bread fruit	6.0
Cactus	6.0
Cantaloupe	7.0
Carob (powdered pod)	5.5
Cherries	5.0
Citron	6.0
Currents	6.0
Dates (dried)	7.0
Fresh	6.0
Figs (dried)	7.0
Fresh	6.0
Gooseberries	6.0
Grapes	6.0
Grapefruit	6.0
Guava	6.0
Kiwi	6.5
Kumquats	6.0
Lemons	7.5
Limes	7.0
Mangos	7.0
Melons (all varieties)	7.0–7.5
Nectarines	6.0
Olives:	
Ripened and sun dried	5.0
Oranges	5.5
Papaya	7.0
Passion fruit	6.5
Peaches	5.5–6.0
Pears	6.0–6.5
Persimmons	6.0
Pineapple	6.5

Pomegranates	5.5
Quince	6.0
Raisins:	
Most all varieties	6.5
Raspberries	5.5
Sapodillas	6.0
Sapote	5.5
Sour grapes	5.5
Strawberries	5.5
Tamarind	6.0
Tangerines	6.0
Umeboshi plums	6.5
Watermelons	7.5

ACID-FORMING

Blueberries	3.5
Cranberries	3.0
If mixed with half water	
Beneficial for bladder and kidney problems	
Plums*	3.5
Prunes*	3.5

VEGETABLES

ALKALINE-FORMING

Artichokes (globe)	4.5
Artichokes (Jerusalem)	5.0
Asparagus	6.5
Bamboo shoots	5.5
Beats	5.5
Broccoli	5.5
Brussels sprouts	5.0
Cabbage	5.5
Carrots	6.0
Cauliflower	5.5
Celery	6.0
Chard, Swiss	6.0
Chicory	5.0

Collards	5.5
Corn, sweet	5.5
Cucumber	5.0
Daikon	5.5
Dandelion greens	6.0
Eggplant	5.0
Endive	6.5
Escarole	6.5
Ginger (fresh)	5.5
Horse radish	4.5
Kale	5.5
Kelp	7.0
Kohlrabi	5.5
Kudzu root (powdered)	7.0
Leeks	5.0
Lettuce:	
Iceberg	5.5
Leaf – all varieties	6.0
Mushrooms	4.5–5.5
Mustard greens	5.5
Okra	5.0
Onion	4.5–5.5

Vidalia onions are sweet and can easily reach the 5.5 range

Onion	
(Spring or scallion)	5.0
Oyster plant	6.0
Parsley	7.0
Parsnips	5.5
Pepper, Bell	5.5
Pickle	5.0

A strong food, use sparingly. Must be prepared with organically grown vegetables, raw, unpasteurized vinegars, and unprocessed salt and spices. All other refined methods of commercial pickling are acid forming 2.0

Potatoes (Irish and sweet)	5.5

Must be eaten with skins otherwise they become acid-forming.

Pumpkin	5.5–6.0

 Depending on variety and sweetness

Radish	5.0

Rhubarb	4.5
Rutabaga	6.0
Salsify	5.5
Sauerkraut	4.5
Seaweed (all types)	7.0

An excellent food

Spinach	6.0
Squash	5.0–6.0

Winter squash rates 5.0. Acorn, butternut, summer, zucchini, and yellow are 6.0. (Raw, organic, yellow squash is high in vitamin B1)

Swiss chard	5.5
Taro (baked)	5.0
Tomatoes	4.5–5.0

Depending on variety and sweetness

Turnips	5.5
Water chestnut (Chinese)	5.0
Watercress	7.0

GRAINS

Acid forming grains become alkaline forming when sprouted and rate 4.5. Those already alkaline forming rate 5.5 when sprouted.

Alkaline-forming

Amaranth	4.5
Millet	4.5
Quinoa	4.5

Acid-forming

Barley	3.0
Basmati rice	2.5
Brown rice	2.5
Buckwheat	2.5
Cornmeal	3.0
Oats (steel cut)	2.5
Rye	3.0
Spelt	3.5
Wheat:	

Whole	2.0
Bleached	1.0

Bleached and radically altered grains are extremely acid-forming. Presume them to be 1.5 at the highest.

White rice (processed)	1.5

No substantial food value. Avoid it.

BEANS
Light proteins

Acid forming dry beans become alkaline forming when sprouted and rate 5.0. Alkaline forming dry soybeans rate 6.0 when sprouted.

Alkaline forming

Green (fresh)	5.5
Lima (fresh)	5.5
Peas (fresh)	5.5–6.0
Snap (fresh)	5.5
Soybean products:	
Dried beans	4.5
Soy cheese	4.5
Soy milk	4.5
Tempeh	4.5
Tofu	4.5
String (fresh)	5.5

Acid-forming

Adzuki	3.5
Black	3.5
Broad beans	3.5
Garbanzo	3.5
Kidney	3.5
Lentils	3.0
Mung	3.5
Navy	3.5
Pinto	3.5
Red	3.5
White	3.5

OTHER STARCHES

Alkaline-forming

Arrowroot	6.0
Cereal	
Granola	4.5
Essene bread	4.5
(Made with sprouted crushed rye and cooked by the sun)	
Potatoes	5.5
(All varieties are alkaline if eaten with the peel)	

Acid-forming

Brans	3.0

Breads
(Refined and cooked at temp. above 300 °F, including all baked flour products such as pancakes, waffles, muffins and pie crusts)

Corn	2.0
Oat	2.0
Rice	2.0
Rye	2.0
Spelt	2.5
Wheat	1.5

Breads
(Organic and cooked at temp. above 300 °F)

Millet	3.0
Corn	2.5
Oat	2.5
Rice	2.5
Rye	2.5
Wheat	2.0

Bread (sprouted and cooked at temp. above 300 °F)

Millet	3.5
Rye	3.0
Wheat	2.5

Cereals (cold)

Unrefined, sweetened with	
honey, maple syrup or fruit.	3.0
Refined,	

artificially sweetened	2.0
Refined, artificially sweetened with preservatives	1.5
Cereals (hot)	
Buckwheat	2.0
Cream of wheat (unrefined)	2.0
Cream of wheat (refined)	1.5
Oatmeal	2.0
Crackers	
Unrefined rye	3.5
Unrefined rice	3.0
Unrefined wheat	3.0
All refined types	2.0
Pastas	
Whole grain with artichoke flour	3.0
Whole grain	2.5
Refined	1.5
Refined with sugar	1.0
Pastries	
Whole grain with honey	2.5
Refined flours with sugar	1.0
Popcorn	
Plain	3.0
With butter	3.0
With salt	2.5
With salt and butter	2.5
Tapioca	2.5

Nuts
Light proteins

Alkaline-forming

Almonds	5.0

Chestnuts (dry roasted)	4.5
Coconut (fresh)	5.0
Pignolias	4.5

Acid-forming

Brazil	3.5
Cashews	3.0
Coconut, dried	3.5
Filberts	3.0
Macadamia	3.0
Peanuts	2.5
Pecans	3.5
Pistachios	3.0
Walnuts	3.0

SEEDS
Light protein

Alkaline-forming

Alfalfa (sprouted)	6.0
Chia (sprouted)	6.0
Radish (sprouted)	5.5
Sesame (not sprouted)	4.5

Acid-forming

Pumpkin	3.0
Sunflower	3.0
Wheat germ	2.0

MEATS
Heavy proteins

- *Canned, chemical and preservative-laden meats drop in value by 0.5*
- *Keep in mind that there are no alkaline-forming meats*

Acid-forming

Bear	1.0
Beef (organically grown)	1.0
Chicken (organically grown)	1.5
Deer	1.5
Fish	
With fins and scales	2.0
The best meat protein	
Other types of fish	1.5
Shell fish	2.0
(Shrimp, scallops, crab, lobster, oysters)	
Goat	1.0
Goat, wild	1.5
Lamb	1.0
Pheasant	1.5
Pork (bacon, barbeque, sausage)	1.0
Rabbit	1.5
Turkey (organically grown)	1.5
Turkey, wild	1.5

ANIMAL PRODUCTS
Light proteins

Neutral or acid forming

Butter:	
Fresh, unsalted	4.0
Fresh, salted	3.5
Processed	3.0
Cheese:	
Mild	3.5
Medium	3.0
Sharp	2.5
Crumbled	3.5

Cow's milk:

Raw	3.5–4.0
Homogenized	3.0
Cream:	
Fresh, raw	4.0
Processed	3.0
Custard:	
With natural ingredients	
With no sugar	3.0
With sugar	2.0
With sugar and preservatives	1.5
Eggs:	
Yolks (coddled, poached, raw or soft boiled)	4.5
Whites	3.5
Whole (fried, scrambled or hard boiled)	2.5
Goat milk:	
Raw	4.5
Homogenized	3.5
Lactobacillus acidophilus	4.0
Lactobacillus bifidus	4.5
Whey	
From cow milk	4.0
From goat milk	4.5
Yogurt	
Plain	4.0
Sweetened	2.0

ANIMAL FATS

<u>Acid-forming</u>

Beef	2.5
Pork	2.0
Lamb	3.0
Chicken	3.0
Fish	3.0

OILS

Neutral and alkaline- forming

Almond	4.0
Avocado	4.0
Canola	4.0
Castor	4.0
Coconut	4.0
Corn	4.0
Margarine	4.0
Olive	4.5
Safflower	4.0
Sesame	4.0
Soy	4.0
Sunflower	4.0

SUGARS

Alkaline-forming

Brown rice syrup	5.0
Dr. Bronner's barley malt sweetener	5.0
Dried sugar cane juice	4.5
Honey	5.0–5.5
Alfalfa, clover, eucalyptus	5.0
Sourwood and tupelo	5.5
Maguey/Agave (Concentrated cactus juice)	5.0

Acid-forming

Artificial sweeteners	0.5
Barley malt syrup	3.0
Beet (processed, bleached)	1.0
Cane (white, processed)	1.0

Iridology Charts

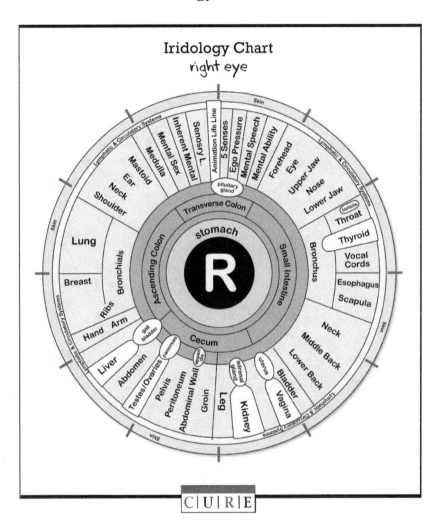

Iridology Chart
right eye

Skin

Lymphatic & Circulatory Systems

Inherent Mental
Senosry L.
Animation Life Line
5 Senses
Ego Pressure
Mental Speech
Mental Ability
Forehead
Eye
Upper Jaw
Nose
Lower Jaw

Mental Sex
Medulla
Mastoid
Ear
Neck
Shoulder

Skin

Lung

Breast

Transverse Colon

pituitary gland

stomach

R

Ascending Colon

Bronchials
Ribs
Hand Arm
Liver
Abdomen

gall bladder

Cecum

pancreas
Testes/Ovaries
Pelvis
Abdominal Wall
appendix
Groin
Leg
adrenal gland
Kidney
uterus
Vagina
Bladder
Lower Back
Middle Back
Neck
Scapula
Esophagus
Vocal Cords
Thyroid
Throat
tonsils
Bronchus
Small Intestine

Lymphatic & Circulatory Systems

Skin

Lymphatic & Circulatory Systems

Skin

Peritoneum

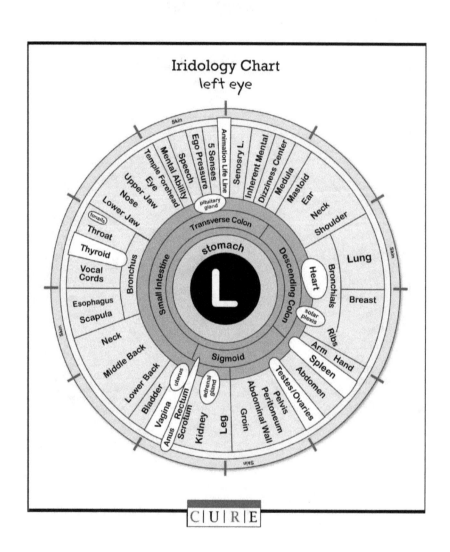

Iridology Chart
left eye

"There is no love sincerer than the love of food."

- **George Bernard Shaw**

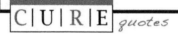

chapter fourteen
Recipes and resources

When it comes to detox food, your focus should be on healing. Taking in fresh and mostly raw cleansing fruits and vegetables will give you the tools you need to detoxify and rejuvenate as rapidly as possible. But of course, most of us really care about flavor and taste along with getting healthy. The goal of these recipes is to deliver health and nutrition along with a side of yummy. These recipes are but a mere sampling of what is available on the internet via blogs, websites, and videos (please see the resource section in this chapter). You must keep in mind a few taboo ingredients during detox when you are surfing the net for more recipe ideas. Just to remind you, they are:

No salt
No black or hot pepper
No oil (of any kind)
No nuts or seeds
No grains or beans
No dairy
No animal protein at all

Once you understand this, the sky is the limit for flavorful raw dishes. There are also a few cooked dishes for those of you who just have trouble breaking away from warm foods, or live in a very cold climate and feel the desire to warm yourself from the inside out.

As you get creative with your meals, keep in mind what makes a particular "dish" a "dish." For example, we could use peppers, onions, and mushrooms twice and end up with two very different meals. If we were to take those ingredients and sauté them in a little bit of water, we could season them either Italian or Mexican-style. For an Italian flair, add garlic, dried oregano, dried basil, and sulfur-free sundried tomatoes. Add this to raw zucchini pasta and you will have a lovely Italian pasta primavera! On the other hand, add cumin, garlic powder, and chili powder, wrap in a collard green and top with fresh guacamole and salsa, and you have a fajita! You see, the same basic ingredients can turn into two totally different meals. It is all about the seasoning. So the next time you crave a dish from your past, think about what makes that dish a dish. The spices and seasonings that your favorite meal featured can be transferred to any number of veggie combinations to bestow them with the flavors you know and love. A Portobello mushroom with homemade raw ketchup, sliced onion, and dill marinated cucumbers between two collard green or cabbage leaves can replace the 4th of July burger that may stare you in the face at your next cookout. Now, as my very Italian mother would say, "mangiare!"

SMOOTHIES

Apple pie smoothie
Makes: 2 Servings
Ingredients:

1 ½	Cups of water
3	Large red delicious apples, chopped
1	Teaspoon pumpkin pie spice
2–4	Tablespoons lemon juice
2	Teaspoons vanilla extract or ½ vanilla bean
	Dash of cinnamon for garnish

Directions:
1. Place all the ingredients in a blender
2. Blend until smooth
3. Top with a dash of cinnamon
4. Let stand for 5 minutes to thicken

Pumpkin smoothie

Makes: 2 Servings
Ingredients:

1	Cup of water
2	Cups fresh grated pumpkin
1 ¼	Teaspoons pumpkin pie spice
6	Medjool dates, pitted
¼	Vanilla bean or 1 teaspoon vanilla extract
4	Ice cubes

Directions:
1. Place all the ingredients in a blender
2. Blend until smooth
3. Adjust spices as desired

Garden smoothie

Makes: 2 Servings
Ingredients:

1	Cup water
1	Cup spinach or kale
1	Tomato, chopped
1	Red bell pepper, seeded and chopped
½	Cucumber, chopped
1	Stalk of celery, chopped
½	The juice from a lemon
1	Small clove of garlic
½	Avocado
	Few Sprigs of your favorite herbs

Directions:
1. Place all the ingredients in a blender
2. Blend until smooth
3. Serve immediately

Cherry-carob smoothie

Makes: 2 Servings
Ingredients:

2	Cups fresh pitted cherries
½	Cup young Thai coconut meat
½	Cup of water
1	Tablespoons carob powder
½	Tablespoon vanilla extract
4	Ice Cubes

A few drops of sweetener of your choice (honey or stevia)

Directions:

1. Place all the ingredients in a blender
2. Blend until smooth
3. Serve immediately

Easy fruit smoothie (This is my favorite because you can use this as a base and add to it as you like. Be sure to follow food combining rules and have fun!)

Makes: 2 Servings

Ingredients:

1–2	oranges
1	inch round of fresh pineapple
1	cup of frozen strawberries
	Then get creative with...
	Peach slices
	Mango
	Cherries
	Kiwi

Directions:

1. Place all the ingredients in a blender keeping the orange closest to the blades
2. Blend until smooth
3. Add ice if desired
4. Serve immediately

Banana smoothie

Makes: 1 Serving

Ingredients:

1	Frozen banana
2–3	dates
	Cinnamon to taste
1	Teaspoons vanilla extract or ½ vanilla bean
	Ice
1	Cup of water

Directions:

1. Place all the ingredients in a blender keeping the banana closest to the blades
2. Blend until smooth
3. Serve immediately

JUICES

Lovely green juice
Makes: 1 Serving
Ingredients:

1	Cucumber
½	Stalk celery
	Equal parts of spinach and kale
1	Green apple
	Several mint leaves
1	Lime

Ultimate green juice
Makes: 2 Servings
Ingredients:

1	Cucumber
½	Stalk celery
10–12	Romaine leaves
1	Cup spinach
	Handful of parsley
1	Green apple of choice

Rainbow juice
Makes: 2 Servings
Ingredients:

1	Apple of choice
1	Beet
2-3	Carrots
½	Stalk celery
1	Cup spinach
	Handful of parsley or cilantro
1	Lemon

BREAKFAST

"Cereal"
Ingredients:
Cereal
¼- ½   Cup of dried mulberries
Toppings:
Sliced organic strawberries
Sliced bananas
Fresh organic blueberries
Organic raisins
(or any other fresh fruit of your choice)
Milk:
1-2   Bananas
1   Cup of water distilled or spring water
(Optional: coconut water instead of distilled or spring water)
(Optional: 1–2 Medjool dates; sprinkle of cinnamon)
As an alternative, you can make fresh coconut milk using the water and meat of a young coconut.
Directions:
1. Place mulberries in a small cereal bowl
2. Top with sliced fruit
3. Add "milk"
4. ENJOY!

Raw apple sauce
Makes: 2 Servings
Ingredients:
2   Apples, peeled and chopped
2   Pitted dates
½   Cup water
Pinch cinnamon, nutmeg, and ginger to taste

Directions:
1. Process in a food processor at medium to high speed until smooth
2. Top with sliced figs, raisins, and/or coconut
3. Serve

Breakfast porridge
Makes: 2 Servings
Ingredients:

1	Pear
1	Banana
1	Apple

Directions:
1. Cut ingredients into chunks
2. Put into blender one by one in order
3. Sprinkle with cinnamon

Peach cobbler
Makes: 2 Servings
Ingredients:

3	Peaches
1	Nectarine or Apricot
2	Pitted Dates
¼	Cup Coconut Flakes

Directions:
1. In a food processor add 2 peaches, dates, and coconut flakes
2. Process until combined (Chunky)
3. Chop up the other peach and nectarine
4. Combine with processed peaches
5. Serve

Stone fruit bowl with dressing
Makes: 2- 4 Servings
Ingredients:
Dressing:

2	tbsp. honey
½	tbsp. Lemon Juice
½	tbsp. Orange Juice
1	tsps. Apple Cider Vinegar

Salad:

1	Peach

1	Plum
½	Cup of cherries pitted
2	Apricots
¼	Cup shredded mint

Directions:
1. Whisk together the dressing ingredients in a small bowl
2. Arrange peaches, plums, cherries, and apricots on plate (Sliced)
3. Drizzle with dressing
4. Garnish with mint
5. Serve

SOUPS, SALADS AND DRESSINGS

Southwest corn chowder
Makes: 4 Servings
Ingredients:

Soup Base:

5	Cups sweet corn kernels; organic; fresh or frozen
2	Cups water
¼	An avocado
3	Garlic cloves
¼	Cup lime juice
½	Teaspoon chipotle powder (typically not used because of its heat, but if aged it can be very mild)

Add-Ins:

1	Diced tomato
½	An avocado
¼	Chopped cilantro

Directions:
1. If fresh corn, carefully remove kernels

2. In a blender, blend 4 cups of corn, water, avocado, garlic, lime juice, and chipotle powder until smooth
3. Stir in additional cup of corn
4. Pour into 4 serving bowls
5. Top with diced tomatoes, avocados, and cilantro
6. Serve

Sancocho suletano
Makes: 6 Servings
Ingredients:

Soup Base:
6	Cups water
3	Cobs Corn cut 1-inch rounds
1	Pounds green plantains peeled and cut
½	Cup diced carrots
½	Cup peas
1	Pound yuca, peeled and cut

Refrito:
1	Tablespoon water
1	Small onion, chopped
2	Garlic cloves

Garnish:
½	Cup chopped cilantro
2	Limes cut into wedges

Directions:
1. In a 4-quart pot, bring water to a boil
2. Add corn, plantains, and carrots
3. Bring back to a rolling boil
4. Lower heat and simmer for 15 minutes
5. While waiting, make refrito
6. Pour water in medium skillet over medium heat
7. Add onion and garlic and sauté for 10 to 12 minutes until onions are soft and slightly brown

8. Add refrito, peas, and yucca to the soup and simmer for another 20 minutes until yuca is soft
9. Ladle the soup into bowls
10. Garnish with sprinkles of cilantro and a lime wedge

Raw vegetable soup
Makes: 1-2 Servings
Ingredients:

1	Zucchini, chopped
2	Stalks of celery, chopped
½	Red bell pepper, chopped
1	Tomato, chopped
1–2	Tsp. lemon, orange or lime juice
Pinch	fresh herbs
1	Chopped Garlic
½–1	Cup water
Pinch	dried seasoning mix of your choice
½	Avocado

Directions:
1. Blend all ingredients except avocado until smooth
2. Add in avocado and blend for a minute
3. Serve

Butternut squash soup
Ingredients:

2	Celery ribs, chopped
1	Carrot, chopped
1	Medium onion, chopped
¼	Teaspoon cinnamon
¾	lb. sweet potatoes
2	Medium Granny Apples peeled
1 ½	lb. Butternut squash, peeled, seeded, and cut into small pieces

2 Cups water

Directions:
1. Heat water in large pot, cook celery, carrot, and onion over low heat until softened

2. While veggies cook, peel potatoes and coarsely chop
3. Core one apple and coarsely chop
4. Stir potato, apple, squash, and water into pot and simmer uncovered, stirring occasionally, until veggies are tender, roughly 15–20 minutes
5. Puree soup in four batches in a blender
6. Return to pot and heat over medium-low heat, stirring until heated through
7. Add water to thin if needed
8. While heating, cut last apple into thin match sticks
9. Serve soup bowls and garnish with apple sticks

Roasted Butternut squash and kale soup

Ingredients:

1	Red, orange or yellow bell pepper, thinly sliced
2	Celery ribs, chopped
2	Carrots, chopped
1	Medium onion, chopped
¼	Teaspoon cinnamon
¾	lb. sweet potatoes
1	Head of kale, stemmed and chopped
1 ½	lb. Butternut squash, whole

2 or more cups water

Directions:

1. Place whole, unpeeled butternut squash on a cookie sheet and place in oven at 400 degrees
2. Allow squash to roast, until it can be easily pierced with a fork. Be sure to pierce the narrow, but denser, area of the squash to be sure it is cooked
3. Once cooked, remove from the oven, carefully cut open and allow to cool
4. In the meantime, in a large pot, add just enough water to cover the bottom of the pot and heat

5. On medium-high heat, add carrots and sweet potatoes. Stir every few minutes and continue to cook for 8 minutes
6. Lower heat to medium. Add bell pepper, onion, celery, and kale and cook for several minutes until all vegetables including potatoes and carrots are tender
7. Once vegetables are cooked, set aside.
8. Scoop seeds out of the butternut squash and discard
9. Scoop meat of butternut squash out of the skin and place in blender with enough water to blend and puree for 30 seconds (Note that the more water used, the thinner the soup will be)
10. Add puree to vegetables and place on medium low heat to mesh the flavors.
11. Remove from heat and sprinkle cinnamon to taste
12. Add water to thin if needed
13. Serve

Chipotle maple dressing
Ingredients:

3	Tablespoons of balsamic vinegar
1 ½	Tablespoons of maple syrup
¼	Teaspoon of chipotle chili powder

Directions:
1. Whisk all ingredients together
2. Pour over salad and toss

Pesto dressing
Ingredients:

1	Avocado
1	Garlic clove, minced

Fresh spinach
Fresh basil
Dried Italian seasoning blend
Cumin to taste

Directions:

1. Place all ingredients in food processor and process until smooth
2. Dressing can be used on salad, as a vegetable dip, on zucchini noodles or on steamed vegetables

Cucumber dill dressing
Ingredients:

1 ½	Cups of cucumbers
1	Garlic clove
1	Teaspoon of lemon juice
½	Avocado
1	Teaspoon of dried dill or a tablespoon of fresh dill, minced

Directions:
1. Place all ingredients except avocado and dill in blender
2. Blend to liquid
3. Add avocado and process until smooth
4. Slow blender and add dill; mix well
5. Enjoy over salad or add more avocado for a vegetable dip

Italian red pepper dressing
Ingredients:

1 ½	Cups of red bell pepper
1	Garlic clove
1	Teaspoon of lemon juice
½	Avocado
1	Teaspoon of dried Italian seasoning

Directions:

1. Place all ingredients except avocado and Italian seasonings in blender
2. Blend to liquid
3. Add avocado and process until smooth
4. Slow blender and add Italian seasoning; mix well
5. Enjoy over salad or add more avocado for a vegetable dip

Classic Dijon honey dressing

Ingredients:

2	Tablespoons of sodium-free Dijon mustard
1	Teaspoon of honey
1	Lemon juiced
2	Tablespoons of apple cider vinegar

2	Tablespoons of water
¼	Teaspoon of fresh thyme
¼	Teaspoon of fresh dill
1	Lavender bloom

Directions:
1. Place all ingredients in a mason jar, screw on lid, and shake
2. Adjust seasonings to taste
3. Will last for one week in refrigerator

Basic dressing

Ingredients:

1	Avocado
1	Clove of garlic, sliced
1 ½- 2	Tablespoons of high quality sulfur-free balsamic vinegar
1	Teaspoon of honey

Directions:

Place all ingredients in blender and blend on low until smooth

Variations of basic dressing choose one of the following and add:

1. Add several leaves of fresh basil; chopped
2. Spicy, brown, or Dijon mustard to taste with a little more honey
3. Roast a red bell pepper, peel the blackened skin and place all ingredients of basic dressing except garlic in a blender and blend; add sliced garlic in last

4. Toss basic dressing with basil with 2–3 fresh diced tomatoes and let marinate for 1 hour- Toss over green salad

Honey dressing
Ingredients:

½ Cup water
½ Avocado
¼ Cup of apple cider vinegar
2 Tablespoons raw honey

Sunny peach salad (Generally frowned upon to mix salad and fruit, but can be done on occasion if there are not digestive issues)
Ingredients:

6 Cups or spring mix (or greens of your choice)
4 Peached, pitted and sliced
¼ Cup of thinly sliced shallot

Directions:
Mix all ingredients and add dressing of choice

Lemon herbs romaine salad
Ingredients and directions:

Hearts of Romaine with creamy avocado, crunchy diced carrots, onion, celery, and tomato. Topped with a light dressing made of fresh squeezed lemon and fresh chopped herbs

Simple, avocado salad
Ingredients and directions:
Diced avocado, celery, tomato and sweet onion. Tossed in a simple mixture of fresh squeezes lime and chopped cilantro. Tangy, creamy and sweet, this salad is perfect over a baked sweet potato.

Whole rainbow salad
Ingredients and directions:

A mix of Romaine lettuce and mixed baby greens. Topped with every vegetable available, including, but not limited to: cucumber slices, daikon and traditional radish, carrot curls, purple cabbage, avocado, sweet onion, tomato, red and yellow bell pepper slices, and sunflower sprouts. Topped with a dressing of your choice.

Crunchy cabbage with honey dressing (see dressings)

Ingredients:
15 cups shredded green cabbage (we used two medium heads, cleaned and cored)
1 bunch (about eight) scallions, finely sliced including some green stems

Directions:
Add honey dressing and toss

Red bell pepper "hummus"
Ingredients:

1	Cup of red bell pepper, chopped
½	Avocado
¼	Cup of fresh lemon juice
2–3	Cloves of garlic
1	Teaspoon of cumin
½	Teaspoon of paprika

Directions:
1. Combine all ingredients in food processor and process until smooth
2. Allow to chill in refrigerator to firm

Entrées

Cauliflower "couscous"
Makes 4 servings
Ingredients:

½	Large head of cauliflower
½	Bunch parsley
¼	Cup fresh mint

2	Diced Roma tomatoes
¼	Red onions chopped
¼	Cup fresh lemon juice
1	Garlic clove, minced
¼	Teaspoon cumin
1/8	Teaspoon smoked paprika

Directions:
1. Chop cauliflower and put in food processor
2. Pulse several times until broken down to the size of rice
3. Transfer to a bowl
4. Put parsley and mint into food processor and pulse until finely chopped
5. Add to cauliflower
6. Stir in remaining ingredients and toss well

Creamy mushroom and eggplant stroganoff
Ingredients:
3	Tbsp. Water
½	Cup diced yellow onion
3–4	Garlic cloves, minced
6	Cups sliced white button and cremini mushrooms
2	Cups homemade vegetable broth or sodium-free broth from the store
1	Eggplant, medium to large
1	Tsp. coconut aminos
1	Tsp. Chopped fresh thyme
2	Zucchini
1	Yellow squash
¼	Cup chopped parsley
2	Tbsp. finely chopped chives

Directions:
1. Remove the eggplant stem, cut in half length wise, and poke skin with fork several times
2. Bake cut side down at 400 degrees for 30 minutes

3. Remove from oven and let cool, then scoop eggplant out of skin
4. Heat 1 tbsp. water in large saucepan over medium-low heat, and sauté the onions till translucent and soft
5. Reduce heat to low and add rest of water, mushrooms, and garlic
6. Sauté on low for 15 minutes, remove from heat
7. Place 1 cup of homemade vegetable stock in blender with roasted eggplant and puree on high for 1 minute
8. Add a cup of the mushroom mixture and pulse till course and grainy, not smooth
9. Pour in saucepan and stir in coconut aminos, thyme, and pepper
10. Place on medium heat and simmer
11. Increase heat slightly after 5 min. and add ½ cup of stock for 10 minutes, cook until thickened
12. Add remaining broth if needed
13. Run the zucchini and squash through a spiralizer and serve stroganoff over zucchini noodles

Portobello mushroom burger
Ingredients:

6	Medium to large Portobello mushrooms
6	Tablespoons balsamic vinegar
	Romaine or collared green leaves for buns
1	Sliced onion
	Broccoli sprouts
1	Serving of guacamole
	Yellow Mustard (sodium-free)
	Sliced tomatoes

Directions:
1. Preheat oven to 350 degrees
2. Wash and de-stem mushrooms in shallow baking dish
3. Place mushrooms gill side up

4. Pour ¼ cup of water into dish
5. Measure 1 tbsp. of balsamic vinegar into the center of each mushroom
6. Make sure to let soak into all the gills
7. Bake for 10 to 12 minutes
8. Build your burger

Five pepper vegetable chili

Ingredients:

Sauce:

1	Cup water
½	Seeded and chopped red bell pepper
3	Tbsp. Sun-dried tomato powder (Make sun-dried tomato powder by grinding sun-dried tomatoes in a spice grinder)
2	Tablespoons orange juice
2	Pitted Medjool dates
1	Tablespoon Mexican chili powder
1	Tablespoon olive oil
1	Garlic clove
½	Teaspoon onion powder
¼	Teaspoon cinnamon

Vegetables:

1	Diced zucchini
1	Diced tomato
1	Organic corn kernels
1	Cup shredded carrots
¼	Diced yellow onion

Directions:
1. Blend all sauce ingredients in blender until smooth
2. Place all veggie ingredients in a large bowl and mix
3. Add sauce to veggies
4. Let stand for 30 minutes (for flavors to blend)
5. Serve

Savory spaghetti squash

Ingredients:

1	Spaghetti squash
¼	Cup vegetable broth
1	Onion, diced
3	Cloves garlic, pressed
1	Green pepper, diced
1	Teaspoon rosemary
1	Teaspoon oregano
1	Teaspoon basil
½	Teaspoon thyme
½	Teaspoon marjoram
1	Tablespoon fresh lemon juice

Directions:
1. Preheat oven to 350 °F
2. Cut squash lengthwise and clean out seeds
3. Place squash cut side down and bake for 45 minutes
4. Remove squash from oven and set aside to cool
5. While squash is baking, sauté onion and garlic in 2 tablespoons vegetable broth in a medium sized skillet over medium heat until onion is soft
6. Add remaining vegetable broth, tomatoes, pepper, spices, and lemon juice
7. Cook for 5-8 minutes
8. Using a fork, gently pull the strands of squash away from the peel, place strands into large serving bowl.
9. Add tomato mixture to squash and mix gently
10. Serve warm

Raw zucchini noodles with raw marinara

Ingredients:

½	Red bell pepper seeded and chopped
2	Tablespoons Sun-dried tomato powder
1–2	Tablespoons water
2	Tablespoons fresh basil
1	Tablespoon fresh oregano

½	Pitted Medjool date
2	Cloves garlic
3	Cups chopped tomatoes

Directions:
1. Blend all except tomatoes in food processor until smooth
2. Add tomatoes and pulse until incorporated but still chunky
3. Spiralize zucchini into ribbons and toss with marina sauce
4. Garnish with diced bell peppers

Scrumptious baked vegetables:
Ingredients:
Baked Vegetables:

1	Medium onion
1	Green bell pepper
1	Sweet potato, cut
1	Head of broccoli, cut
½	lb. mushrooms
1	Pint cherry tomatoes, halved
1	Medium zucchini, sliced
	Garlic powder
	Onion powder

Sauce:

¼	Cup balsamic vinegar
¼	Cup maple syrup
1	Tablespoon freshly squeezed orange juice
1	Teaspoon thyme, dried
1	Teaspoon basil, dried
1	Teaspoon rosemary, dried
1	Garlic clove, minced

Desserts

Pumpkin pie:
Ingredients:
Crust:

| 2 | Cups dried coconut |

1	Cup pitted dates
1/8	Teaspoon cinnamon

Filling:

3	Cups butternut squash, shredded
1	Cup pitted dates
1	Tablespoon vanilla extract
1	Tablespoon of Pumpkin spice
½	Cup organic apple sauce
1	Cup coconut water

Raw vegan candy balls

Ingredients:

1	cup pitted dates
½	cup shredded coconut

Directions:
1. Combine in food processor using S blade
2. Process until mixture becomes a ball
3. Mold into desired shapes

Orange truffles:

Ingredients:

1	Cup pitted Medjool dates
2	Tablespoons orange juice
2	Tablespoons orange zest
1/8	Teaspoon vanilla powder or ½ teaspoon vanilla extract
1	Tablespoons carob powder

Directions:
1. Place all ingredients except cacao in food processor and process until well combined
2. Scoop out one heaping tablespoon at a time and roll into balls
3. Sprinkle cacao powder onto flat clean surface and roll until coated
4. Shake off excess carob powder
5. Serve immediately or chilled to firm up

Resources

Because this is a book and not a webpage, the information regarding resources is only up to date at the date of the printing. For this reason, I am going to include the web address of my practice so that you can go there for information regarding new movies, recipes, videos etc.

I will also include the current resources that we share with our patients.

http://www.partnersinhealing.org/Resources.html

Recipes:
http://www.partnersinhealing.org/Breakfast.pdf
http://www.partnersinhealing.org/Juices___Smoothies.pdf
http://www.partnersinhealing.org/Entr__es.pdf
http://www.partnersinhealing.org/Salads.pdf
http://www.partnersinhealing.org/Desserts.pdf
http://www.partnersinhealing.org/Soups.pdf

Inspiring documentaries:
These documentaries can be found in numerous places like Amazon.com, NETFLIX, youtube.com, as well as the websites of individual producers of the films. Google search and enjoy!

Food Matters
Fat, Sick, and Nearly dead
Eating
Forks over Knives
Simply Raw
The Gerson Miracle
Food Inc.
Vegucated
Hungry for Change
Earthlings
Supersize Me

The Beautiful Truth
Diet for a New America
Meet Your Meat
Processed People
Farmageddon
Dying to Have Known
Fed Up
Juicing Saved My Life
Cowspiracy
Healing Cancer from the Inside Out

Books
The Secret Life of Plants by Christopher Bird
The Detox Miracle Sourcebook by Robert Morse ND
Raw Vegetable Juices by Dr. N.W. Walker
Fresh Vegetable and Fruit Juices by Dr. N.W. Walker

Online stores and safe products
In recommending these websites, please keep in mind that a vast majority of the products found there are *not detoxification-friendly*. But they are still a great resource for things like sulfite-free, dried fruit, natural body-care products, and toxic-free home cleaning products as well as more natural choices in pet supplies. While I have found preparing fresh meals for my dog to be the absolute best choice for his health, it is not always financially feasible or timely to do so. Therefore, having a resource that you can trust has proven to be a good balance.
http://www.nuts.com
Gohealthypet.com
Vitacost.com
https://www.facebook.com/PrimalPitPaste/?hc_location=ufi
http://www.sujajuice.com/
https://www.doterra.com/en
http://www.kuumbamade.com/store/index.php?p=home
My favorite juice extractors: **https://www.omegajuicers.com/**
My favorite blender (I have had the same blender for 23+ years): **https://www.vitamix.com/**

Paint
http://www.mythicpaint.com.hk/file/en/
http://www.ecosimplista.com/

Cranial sacral therapy
*Upledger institute: **http://www.upledger.com/***

Lymphatic drainage
http://www.therapeuticflow.org/

Meditation
http://www.vipassana.com/
http://www.vipassanadhura.com/

Acupuncture Physicians
http://www.nccaom.org/

Chiropractors
http://www.acatoday.org/

Emotional Freedom Technique (EFT)
http://www.emofree.com/eft-tutorial/tapping-basics/what-is-eft.html

Detoxification information
At Partners in Healing we are happy to take your calls or emails. Please visit our website for more information.
www.partnersinhealing.org
letnatureheal.blogspot.com
http://letnatureheal.blogspot.com/2012/03/true-healing-and-end-of-graves-disease.html
https://www.youtube.com/watch?v=myoiZti3mB0

Homemade vegetable washes

2 cups of cold tap water, 1/4 cup of white vinegar, and 2 tablespoons lemon juice

Mix these ingredients well together and pour into a spray bottle. Squirt your produce 2–3 times, let it rest for two minutes, and then rinse off with more tap water before consuming.

or

1 cup of cold fresh water, 1/2 cup of white vinegar, 1 tablespoon lemon juice, and 1/8 teaspoon grapefruit seed extract

This next way to wash looks similar to the first, but also contains just a hint of grapefruit seed extract, a known antioxidant with possible antimicrobial properties. Shake everything together in a spray bottle once again, and apply, let sit, and rinse.

or

1 cup water, 1 tablespoon lemon juice, and 1 tablespoon baking soda

Swap out vinegar for baking soda for a foamy alternative. Spray on veggies and let them rest for five minutes, before rinsing and patting dry.

or

1/2 cup water, 1/2 cup vinegar, 2 tablespoons salt

This mixture is more concentrated than the others, and should be used as a half-hour soak for some serious fruit n' veg cleansing. Salt helps draw out bugs and other nasties hiding in leafy green veggies, while the vinegar vanquishes them!

"Knowing yourself is the beginning of all wisdom."

- Aristotle

C|U|R|E *quotes*

chapter fifteen
Self-assessment survey

Thyroid/Parathyroid (Glandular System)

Yes No Are you overweight?

Yes No Do you get cold hands and feet?

Yes No Do you have hair loss, are you bald, or going bald?

Yes No Is it easy to put on weight and hard to lose it?

Yes No Are your fingernails ridged, brittle, or weak?

Yes No Do you have varicose or spider veins?

Yes No Do you have, or have you ever had hemorrhoids?

Yes No Do you get cramping in your muscles?

Strong Weak Is your bladder strong or weak?

Yes No Do you have an irregular heartbeat?

Yes No Do you have Mitral Valve Prolapse (*Heart Murmur*)?

Yes No Do you get headaches or migraines?

Yes No Do you now have, or have you ever had a hernia?

Yes No Have you ever had an aneurysm?

Yes No Do you have osteoporosis?

Yes	No	Do you have scoliosis?
Yes	No	Do you get irritable easily?
Yes	No	Do you have low energy levels?
Yes	No	Do you suffer from symptoms of depression?
Yes	No	Did you score low on your bone density tests?
Yes	No	Do your tests come back showing low Calcium levels?
Yes	No	Do you have, or have you ever had a goiter?
Yes	No	Do you have spine deterioration or herniated discs?
Yes	No	Have you been diagnosed with Hashimoto's or Reidel's disease?
		(Or any family member?)
A lot	A little	Do you sweat profusely or hardly at all?

Adrenal Glands (Glandular System)
Medulla (Adrenal)

Yes	No	Do you have M.S., Parkinson's or Palsy?
Yes	No	Do you have anxiety attacks or feel overly anxious?
Yes	No	Do you feel excessive shyness, or inferior to others?
Yes	No	Do you have low blood pressure (below 118 systolic)?
Yes	No	Do you have tremors, nervous legs, etc.?
Yes	No	Do you have tinnitus (ringing in the ears)?
Yes	No	Do you have S.O.B. (shortness of breath) or is it hard to take a deep breath?

Yes	No	Do you have heart arrhythmias?
Yes	No	Do you have a hard time sleeping?
Yes	No	Do you have Chronic Fatigue Syndrome?
Yes	No	Do you get tired easily?
Yes	No	Have you ever been diagnosed with Addison's Disease or Congenital Adrenal Hyperplasia?

Cortex (Adrenal)

Yes	No	Do you have elevated blood cholesterol levels?
Yes	No	Do you have lower back weakness?
Yes	No	Do you have, or have you had sciatica?
Yes	No	Do you have arthritis or bursitis?
Yes	No	Do you have any "itis' (inflammatory conditions)?

Female only

Yes	No	Are your menstruations irregular?
Yes	No	Do you get excessive bleeding during menstruation?
Yes	No	Do you have or have you had ovarian cysts?
Yes	No	Do you have or have you had fibroids?
Yes	No	Do you have or did you have endometriosis or A-typical cells?
Yes	No	Are you fibrocystic?
Yes	No	Do you have fibromyalgia or scleroderma?
Yes	No	Do you get sore breasts, especially during menstruation?

Yes	No	Do you have a low or excessive sex drive?
Yes	No	Have you had a hysterectomy?

Partial _____ *Complete* _____

Yes	No	Did they remove any other organs at the same time? (*ex. gallbladder)*
Yes	No	Have you had a D & C?
Yes	No	Have you had a miscarriage?
Yes	No	Have you had difficulty in conceiving children?

Male Only

Yes	No	Do you have prostatitis (*frequent urination esp. at night*)?

If yes, how often?

Yes	No	Do you have prostate cancer? PSA count _____
Yes	No	Do you have testicular hypertrophy (*enlargement*)?
Yes	No	Do you have a low or excessive sex drive?
Yes	No	Do you have erection problems?
Yes	No	Do you have premature ejaculation?

Pancreas

Yes	No	Do you get gas after you eat?
Yes	No	Do you feel your foods just sitting in your stomach?
Yes	No	Do you have acid reflux?
Yes	No	Do you see any undigested foods in your stools?

Yes	No	Do you have hypoglycemia (*Low Blood Sugar*)?
Yes	No	Do you have Diabetes (*High Blood Sugar*)?
		Type I ___ or Type II ___
Yes	No	Are you thin and have a hard time putting on weight?
Yes	No	Do you have gastritis or enteritis?
Yes	No	Do your foods pass right through you (*diarrhea*)?
Yes	No	Do you have moles on your body?

Skin

Yes	No	Do you get or have skin rashes?
Yes	No	Do you get skin blemishes?
Yes	No	Do you have Eczema or Dermatitis?
Yes	No	Do you have Psoriasis?
Yes	No	Do you itch anywhere? Where?
Yes	No	Is your skin dry?
Yes	No	Is your skin excessively oily?
Yes	No	Do you get or have dandruff?

Gastro-Intestinal Tract

Yes	No	Is your tongue coated (white, yellow, green or brown), especially in the morning?
Yes	No	Do you have a Hiatus Hernia?
Yes	No	Do you have Gastritis?
Yes	No	Do you have Enteritis?

Yes	No	Do you have Colitis?
Yes	No	Do you have Diverticulitis?
Yes	No	Do you get or have diarrhea?
Yes	No	Do you get or have constipation?
Yes	No	How often do you have a bowel movement?
Yes	No	Have you ever had stomach or intestinal ulcers?
Yes	No	Do you or have you ever had any type of gastro-intestinal cancers:
Yes	No	stomach, colon, rectal, etc.
		Explain:
Yes	No	Do you have Crohn's Disease?
Yes	No	Do you have "gas" problems?
Yes	No	Other GI problems:

Liver/Gallbladder/Blood

Yes	No	Do you have a problem digesting fats?
Yes	No	Do fats or dairy foods cause bloating and/or pain in the stomach area?
Yes	No	Is your stool white or very light brown in color?
Yes	No	Do you get pain in the middle of your back (especially after eating)?
Yes	No	Do you get pain behind the right lower rib area?
Yes	No	Do you have "liver" or brown spots on your skin (Not freckles)?
Yes	No	Do you have any skin pigmentation changes?
Yes	No	Do you have skin problems? If so, what type?

Yes   No   Are you anemic?

Yes   No   Do you have, or have you ever had hepatitis?
A___, B___, C___.

Heart & Circulation

Yes   No   Do you have any gray hair?

Yes   No   Do you have a hard time remembering things?

Yes   No   Do your legs get tired or cramped after you walk?

Yes   No   Do you bruise easily?

Yes   No   Do you get chest pains or angina?

Yes   No   Have you ever had a heart attack (Myocardial Infarction)?

Yes   No   Have you ever had open-heart surgery?

Yes   No   Do you have heart arrhythmias?

Yes   No   What kind?

Yes   No   Do you have a heart murmur or Mitral Valve Prolapse?

Yes   No   Do you ever feel pressure on your chest?

Yes   No   Do you get "prickly" pains anywhere, especially in the heart area?

Where?_____

Yes   No   Do you have, or have you ever had High Blood Pressure?

Yes   No   Your average blood pressure is _____ over _____

Lymphatic System

Yes   No   Are you allergic to anything? What?

Yes   No   Do you ever get colds or flu-like symptoms?

Yes No Do you have sinus problems?

Yes No Do you have or get sore throats?

Yes No Do you have swollen lymph nodes?

Yes No Do you have or had tumors? What type?
Fatty___ Benign___ Cancerous
Where?_____

Yes No Do you have a low platelet count (blood)?

Yes No Is your immune system low or sluggish?

Yes No Have you had appendicitis or an appendectomy?
When?

Yes No Do you get boils, pimples, and the like?

Yes No Do you have allergies?

Yes No Have you ever had abscesses?

Yes No Have you ever had toxemia?

Yes No Do you have, or have you had, cellulitis?

Yes No Have you ever had gout?

Yes No Do you get blurred vision?

Yes No Do you have mucus in your eyes when you wake up in the morning?

Yes No Do you snore?

Yes No Do you have sleep apnea?

Yes No Have you had your tonsils out? What age? _____

Kidneys

Yes No Have you ever had a urinary tract infection (UTI's)?

Yes No Have you ever had "burning" upon urination?

Yes No Do you have bags under your eyes (esp. in the morning)?

Yes No Is your urine flow restricted?

Yes No Do you get cramping or pain on either side of your mid-to-lower back?

Yes No Do you or did you ever have nephritis?

Yes No Do you or did you ever have cystitis?

Lungs

Yes No Do you get or have (or have had) bronchitis?

Yes No Do you get or have (or have had) emphysema?

Yes No Do you get or have (or have had) asthma?

Yes No Do you get or have (or have had) C.O.P.D?

Yes No Are you on inhalers or nebulizers? How often?

Yes No What type?

Yes No Do you know what your oxygen saturation is _____?

Yes No Do you get pain when you breathe?

Yes No Do you get pain when you take a deep breath?

Yes No Did you ever or do you have lung cancer?

Yes No Do you have a collapsed lung?

Yes No Are you a smoker? How often?

Yes No Have you ever had pneumonia?

Yes No Have you ever worked around toxic chemicals, in coal mines or around asbestos?

Yes No Do you cough a lot?

Yes No Do you get any mucus when you cough?

Yes No What color is the mucus?

*"And in the end the love you take
is equal to the love you make."*

- John Lennon/Paul McCartney

C|U|R|E *quotes*

chapter sixteen
Final Words

Before moving forward, it is very important to address the fact that not all situations are able to be reversed. There are extenuating circumstances that stand in the way of healing. These circumstances include, but are not limited to:

- A high level of toxicity due to poisons, medications, chemotherapy, radiation, etc.

- A very weak body that has been sick for an extended period of time

- Severe genetic weakness

- A spirit's time to move on

- I cannot care more about your health than you do

Where do we go from here?

A patient once asked me "is detox ever truly over?" As you could imagine the answer is quite complex. I might start with "have you reached your health goals?" But there are other things to consider.

- How long have you been dealing with this particular health issue?

- Do you have any other health concerns beside the primary one?

- What do your eyes say? Is there a great deal of lymphatic congestion or genetic weakness as seen in your iridology photos?

- How many years have you lived a toxic lifestyle?

- What got you here and how important is it for you to never return to this toxic state?

While the detoxification protocol may be finished, our goal should ALWAYS be to avoid that toxic state in the future. In plain English, do not return to the habits that caused your illness, weakness, and acid state. You must find a balance in your life that will allow you to maintain an optimal state of health and vitality while being able to live in the "real world." That does not mean that you give into others' definition of the real world. It means you create your world so that you can coexist with others who are not on this path.

I personally have not ventured too far away from my clean, detox diet for several reasons. The most important reason is that I feel amazing eating this way! As you step back into the non-detox arena (if you are listening), your body will tell you exactly what works and what does not. I have taken many a phone call, email, or text where a detox graduate "celebrated" the normalization of a blood test or shrinking of a tumor with an all-American meal, a ½ bottle of wine or ice cream cake…or all three! These grand celebrations are usually followed by abdominal pains, flu-like symptoms, headaches, or even skin rashes. It is my hope that my patients celebrate this "negative" reaction in their body and not be upset by it. A reaction to toxins is something your body was inhibited from in the past due to years of suppression. In other words, the more toxins you put in your body over the years, the less ability the body had to react. It just couldn't.

If your body reacted to every toxic or acidic food you ate, cream you rubbed on to your skin, or chemical cleaner you inhaled, it would be in a state of constant upheaval. Instead, the body moves these toxins to a place where it can deal with them later (fat cells and lymph). In essence, it prioritizes. Eventually, the stored toxins affect the cells around them and, well you know the rest. So why then, after all of this cleaning and detoxing do we have a reaction to the burger, wine, or ice cream? Look at it this way…

If you visited the Ohio River (known as one of the most polluted rivers in the United States) and poured a can of motor oil into it, you would be hard-pressed to notice it. In some areas of the Ohio River, the waters are so dirty, it is impossible to make a distinction between newly added waste and the contamination which already exists. But, if you took that same can of motor oil and drove to the mountains of Vermont and then poured it into a pristine brook, stream or river, you would immediately notice the thick, black sludge. This, my friends, is the state of the body before and after detox. Now that you are clean(er) it is far easier to notice the toxicity of the "food" that you put into your body. As I've stated in previous chapters, it is not that you will never again have a slice of pizza or birthday cake. However, please take note of how your body feels after consuming more acid food and make a decision as to how often you are willing to go there. Keep in mind, with your newfound knowledge and the endless resources on the internet, you can make ice cream, pizza and cake in a much healthier manner.

On your post detox diet, variety abounds and all it takes is a sense of adventure and curiosity! Let's start with some basic guidelines.

Acid/Alkaline balance

As you recall, during the detoxification process, you were on 100% alkaline-forming foods. This is the only way to reverse the course of disease and keep you on the alkaline side of chemistry. Once detoxification is over, it is strongly advised that you consume 80% (or more) alkaline foods and 20% (or less) acid-forming foods. In a side note, it is very important to understand that all alkaline food still has an acid component. Fruit and vegetables are "alkaline-dominant" yet they are not void of acidic aspects. So whether you are on a detox diet or post-detox diet, you WILL NEVER BE TOO ALKALINE!

Some people make the decision to not remain vegan, please follow these important concepts.
- Do not eat more than 8oz. of animal protein each week.

- Be sure that the animal protein sources that you consume are free-range, grass fed, and organic.

- Do not consume milk or milk products of any kind.

- Avoid "bottom-feeders" from the ocean and instead choose deep water fish.

If you would like to increase the amount of protein in your diet, you can follow Anthony's post detox meal plan (see Chapter 4: "Where do you get your protein?"). Of course you must ask yourself your reason for increasing protein levels in your diet. Are you doing so because you feel pressure from others? Do you believe your body will be healthier? Or are you looking to increase skeletal muscle? The truth is you need much less protein than you think in order to build muscle size and strength. The reason for this goes back to, you guessed it, acid! If you have been a serious weight lifter, know people who are, or read a lot of fitness magazines, you probably are aware of the diets of such individuals. You know that during detoxification, dietary protein is greatly restricted in an effort to reduce stress on the kidneys, allowing them to focus on filtering stagnant acid waste. Once detox is over, many people believe that they have to "build up" again by increasing protein significantly. But, if they understood what I call the "protein cycle" they would see things differently.

For all those who eat a high protein diet to build muscle, an interesting phenomenon occurs. At first a weight lifter may increase protein by adding an egg to their oatmeal breakfast. Lunch may include a tuna sandwich while dinner is some vegetables and baked chicken breast. Off to the gym they go every morning to pound some weights, stopping at Subway to pick up lunch and the local fast-food rotisserie restaurant to pick up dinner. Sure they begin to get some muscle growth, but soon they discover that their growth plateaus and may even reverse. So what do they do? They increase their protein intake of course! Two eggs at breakfast, a whole can of tuna for lunch, an afternoon whey-protein shake and two chicken breasts for dinner. This is coupled with a second weight lifting session in the evening. Eventually cardiovascular workouts such as running or the elliptical machine are eliminated to avoid "burning up" muscle and once again a plateau or reduction in muscle size leads to another increase in dietary protein. Why do we see this cycle over and over? Why does muscle stagnate or diminish if the diet contains such high amounts of protein? The answer is simple. Dietary protein such as eggs, tuna, chicken breast, and whey protein are all extremely acidic. And what does acid do? It destroys tissue, ALL tissue, including the muscle that it was supposed to support. That is why the weightlifting and body building industry is such a lucrative business. They destroy the tissue which they claim to build, leaving you with no alternative but to continuously up the ante of protein shakes, bars and supplements.

However, if you keep your protein as alkaline as possible you will find that you can build and maintain strength as well as muscle mass without the steady increase of protein.

On a side note, you should ask yourself, "What is my end goal?" Is it size, strength or optimal health? The answer should be obvious. Optimal health always trumps size and strength. Of course we all want to be strong enough to carry on activities from sports to lifting heavy boxes to lifting ourselves off of the toilet when we are 80. But excess "strength" in the form of gargantuan muscles actually weakens other parts of the body, like bones, organs and glands. The amount of protein required to build large, disproportionate muscles for our frame ultimately leads to an acid state and you know where an acid state takes you.

Here are some of the foods to incorporate.
- Raw organic walnuts—a wonderful source of vegan protein with a low incidence of allergies. I find that cashews and almonds, which are more commonly used in raw vegan diets, tend to congest the sinus, mucus membranes of the respiratory and digestive tracts as well as cause bloating more than walnuts. It is my personal experience that walnuts when eaten in moderation, are well-tolerated.
- Raw sunflower seeds

- Raw pumpkin seeds

- Raw sesame seeds

- Raw hemp seed

- Raw chia seeds

- Quinoa–technically a fruit but eaten as a grain

- Beans that are green in color and can be eaten raw. This includes green or "string" beans.

- Sprouts–sunflower, alfalfa, pea, bean.

- Spinach

Honestly, do not overthink protein. Follow Chapter 4 and enjoy real, whole food.

Grains

If you venture into the nutrition section of the book store, you are immediately struck with the enormity as well as variety of books on the shelves. We have been through the low sugar craze, low fat fad and these days, low carbs trend. There is a great deal of information about how carbohydrates, mainly grains and products made from them contribute significantly to American's weight issues. Yes, we see that for many individuals, removing grain from the diet often times results in weight loss. And while excess weight is certainly a contributing factor to many diseases, I have another reason why grains should only be reintroduced in the diet in small amounts. Of course, if you choose to leave them out of your diet after detoxification is over, I am fine with that as well.

I generally feel that grains are difficult to digest. In ancient Chinese medicine, practitioners would prescribe congees for various digestive and other ailments. Congees are usually made from rice or another grain and cooked for many hours with a lot of water or some type of broth. The rice and liquid seemingly become "one" rendering it much easier to digest. But it takes long term slow cooking to break down the fiber of the grain to make it more easily digestible. My belief is that if something has to be cooked for that long to make it usable by the body, I'd rather stick to fresh fruit and vegetables. On a different note, grains, especially those containing the protein "gluten," have a way of gluing up the intestines, reducing our ability to absorb nutrition from food.

What then is the bottom line when it comes to grain? Follow these basic guidelines:

- Choose grains that do not contain gluten: Millet, quinoa, brown rice, buckwheat, amaranth, teff and montina (Indian rice grass).

- Eat these grains and products made from them in their "whole grain form."

- Consume grains in no more than one meal a day and no more than three days a week. There are so many "non-grain" products out there to substitute that you will always have variety. There are even grain-free wraps such as SunFood Superfoods Raw Vegan Coconut Wraps.

- Be conscious! If you eat grains a few times a week and you have no digestive issues, skin issues, sinus congestion etc. great! If you do have responses to grains, stay away from them or keep them at a minimum.

Oils/fats

Oils can be controversial in that raw vegans prefer avoiding processed oils like coconut, olive, almond etc. Yet we understand that the body requires fats for such functions as absorbing other nutrients, producing hormones, maintaining skin and other tissue as well as for optimal brain function. But consuming highly processed fat can be likened to consuming high fructose corn syrup. Oils are typically heated (even cold-pressed generally must be heated to deal with contaminants from the extraction process) which has been thought to alter their molecular structure which can contribute to cancer. As an Italian, I was raised with olive oil. In fact, I am quite sure that if I cut a vein, olive oil would pour out! I know you are looking for a definitive answer and at this point in my research and physical experience, I cannot provide you with one. I can only tell you what I have observed.

These days, if I eat a cooked meal that has been prepared with oil, I can almost certainly feel its effects the next day. I may wake up in the morning with some mucus in my throat, or the need to blow my nose. I might feel a bit sluggish or have a strong urge to use the bathroom. I chalk this up to my body's level of hygiene and its willingness to remove anything that might hinder optimal health. Does that mean I will never consume a cooked meal or processed oil? No. I live in this world with friends and family who do not necessarily eat or live the way I do. Sometimes, by the end of the work week, I like to go out to a restaurant with my husband, sit outside and chat while eating some Thai food. During the holidays, I pull out my raw food books or Google a vegan holiday recipe and create a festive meal. I will certainly never give up a clean life-style and go backwards. But I am also not willing to live in a bubble. Our bodies were created with an incredible ability to cleanse and regenerate itself. I certainly do not feel that we are fragile. After breaking my pelvis when falling off my horse, some friends inquired as to whether I would give up riding. "Given the risks involved," they said, "wouldn't it be smart to stop?" I chose to continue riding. This is life my friends, and I do not want to see you or me living in such a restrictive manner as to not experience all of the joys it has to give. For without darkness there is no light. However, I also want you to refer back to the chapter on consciousness. Whether choosing your meals, your activities, or your friends, it is wise to make all decisions with consciousness. That being said, here are some guidelines.

- Oil should be obtained first from the consumption of raw nuts and seeds as well as ripe avocado. Do not go overboard. Start slowly and observe changes in digestion, mucus, congestion, joint or body pain, etc. Listen to your body!

- When consuming processed oil, be sure to find the best oils possible. First cold pressed and cloudy. Yes, I said cloudy! The cloudier the oil is (I have seen some amazing bottles of olive oil that where so cloudy, I could hardly see through them) the less refined it is.

- Add oil to a raw dish or after it has been cooked for flavor. Whenever my husband is in the mood for a "stir-fry", I will water sauté the veggies using garlic, onion and ginger (and usually some type of hot pepper) and then add some sesame oil for flavor at the very end. Using oil in this way will reduce the amount used and maintain full flavor.

- If you do choose to heat oil for cooking, it is generally recommended that you use oils that can stand up to heat. Traditionally oils with high smoke points, such as corn, soybean, peanut and sesame, are suggested for high-heat frying and stir-frying. I am not a fan of corn, soybean or peanut oil. Sesame oil is the best option. Olive, canola, and grapeseed oils have moderately high smoke points, which makes them a better choice for sautéing over medium-high heat. Oils with low smoke points, such as flaxseed and walnut, are best saved for use in salad dressings and dips.

- Remember to pay attention, be conscious, and listen to your body. It will tell you what works and what does not.

Salt

During detoxification added salt is removed from the diet. Of course, naturally occurring sodium supplied by vegetables provides the body with all that is needed for functions such as muscle contraction, nerve conduction and blood pressure regulation. However, Americans consume over 1000 mg more salt per day than what is recommended by the US Department of Health and Human Services (DHHS). I feel that the DHHS recommendations are too high if we follow the basic premise from our species conversation so many chapters ago.

Sodium is a necessity of life, but by the time you complete your 8, 10, or 50 week detox you will be pleasantly surprised at how little you miss it. Once off of a detox diet, it is easy to rapidly increase your sodium intake. Restaurant foods, condiments like ketchup, mustard, salad dressing or hot sauce contain tremendous amounts of added salt, much of which is iodized and demineralized leading to imbalances in the body's pH, dehydration, and water retention.

Have I depressed you yet? That is certainly not my intention. Do you notice a trend happening in this chapter? If you don't, you should. The trend here is twofold.
1. I will not tell you what you should or should not eat. I will not make you "wrong."

2. Consciousness. In consciousness YOU will decide what works for you and what does not.

My acupuncture practice is called Partners in Healing for a reason. Your input, say, and decisions are just as important as mine. As they say, when the teacher is ready the student will come. So too, when the student is ready, the teacher will come. It is time for you to become the teacher. Go out and help others to learn what you have learned. But you can only do this when you step into conscious awareness and there is no better way to do so post-detox. Post detox is the time when you can really understand what your food choices had been doing to your body. As our health improves, we tend to forget the physical issues that plagued us. Our energy returns, headaches go away and skin clears up. It is not until the post-detox state that we experience toxins on an immediate level. As you observe what works and what does not in your body, I challenge you to find joy in the process and turn your back on sorrow. Instead of complaining about what you can't eat, revel in the doors that have been open to you and seek out new foods to enjoy. (The good news is that there are many recipes on the internet for homemade condiments that taste better and contain little to no salt.) Add a little salt, some pepper and oil. Play with your food. But also realize that the journey is not over and that is a good thing!

Alcohol, coffee and other detox no-nos

Ah yes, I knew this day would come. The day I had to put in writing my views on this magic elixir! Truth be told, I never really drank much. After high school, I spent one spring break at night clubs dancing and drinking very watered-down rum and Cokes. When my best friend and I moved out of our parents' homes for the first time, we purchased a six pack of wine coolers and got wasted in our back yard! Years later, in fire college, my classmates and I looked forward to Friday afternoon when we turned our uniform shirts inside out and headed to the park to guzzle down a couple of cold beers on ice. It was summer-time in Florida, the temperature was 95 °F and a cold beer went down quickly and easily.

Those were really the only times in my life I drank with any significance. Today, we read about the benefits of wine, beer, and other forms of alcohol as they are touted for their antioxidant value, ability to help diabetes (I can't wrap my head around that one either), fight colds, or burn fat. All I can tell you, is if you have a lot of extra time on your hands, please investigate *who paid for those studies.* It is likely that the author of the study stood a good chance to benefit from writing a glowing review of those intoxicating spirits.

If you are looking for a way to fight colds, burn fat or prevent heart disease, you found it in Chapters 1–10 of this book! Am I saying never have another glass of wine? No more than I am saying never have another piece of birthday cake. But you have worked diligently, put in mountains of effort and reaped unheard of benefits. If you choose to celebrate with wine, beer, or a Margarita (in the words of my mentor, Dr. Morse) "you can, *but...*" you don't want to make a habit of it.

My husband, Anthony was a coffee-a-holic. He woke with espresso, snacked on espresso and followed dinner with, you guessed it, espresso. Several years before detox he decided to quit drinking it cold turkey. Anthony experienced headaches and nausea for about two days. Then it was over. These days he drinks a cup of dark roast coffee about 1–2 times a week. He calls it a "dessert item." I personally never liked coffee so it was never an issue for me. But many people around the world live for their coffee. The question I always ask, of course, is why?

Why are we addicted to coffee? Is it the taste or more likely what is does for us? Coffee gets us up and gets us going. In fact, I have a friend that cannot even get up in the morning without it. He remains in bed while his wife makes coffee and brings in to him. It is not until he has had two cups that he can get out of bed and start his day. If you were drinking coffee to get you going and give you energy, don't worry, detox will fix that. You will be endowed with boundless energy once you have completed detox. So why would you choose to go back to coffee after detox? Is it because of the antioxidant benefits? (If so, don't worry, fruit provides the same if not more benefits.) Do you need to drink coffee or just want to?

If you want to drink coffee, I caution you to limit the amount you drink. As you know, it is highly addictive AND highly acidic. Don't go down that rabbit hole. Instead think about following Anthony's lead and have it as an occasional treat. Then you can really appreciate the taste and occasion.

A final note about reintroducing non-detox food.

I am certain after reading this book, you have grown accustomed to my love of analogies. In an effort to not disappoint, here is another one. When you reintroduce any food to your freshly cleaned body and you have a reaction to it, I would like you to think about a baby. When a baby is born into the world, she has come from a relatively pristine environment. Mom has nurtured and protected her within the womb and now begins the job of nourishing her with breast milk. After a period of time, mom may decide to return to work and will have to "pump" milk so that the baby can be fed while she is away. After some time, pumping may become inconvenient and commercial formula is introduced. Over a few days or maybe a few weeks the baby may become fussy, not sleep through naps or the night, develop colic, "catch a cold," or develop eczema. At her next checkup the parents question the pediatrician about these changes and the doctor replies with the standard answers..." babies get colic; maybe someone around you had a cold; babies develop eczema—we don't know why."

These standard answers are not answers, they are statements of occurrences but they do not prove cause or provide a solution. Meanwhile no one questions the obvious...diet change. This brand new pristine body has been given "food" that provides some semblance of nutrition, but it is not "clean" to the body and the body responds, sometimes mildly and sometimes with great aversion! So too might your body after detox. It may see some food as toxic or irritating. You see, you have become clean and new (maybe not as clean or new as a tiny baby, but you get the point)! If you continue to eat irritating food, there is a good chance your body will eventually stop reacting to it, much like it did all those years ago, before you decided to detox. You will have to make the decision as to how much and how often you want to eat something. It is all in your hands, grasshopper! Take what you have learned from your body and apply it wisely.

Revisiting detoxification in the future

Finally, the questions of "am I done? Am I fixed? Am I CURED?" The answer to these questions lies within you. Again, the same questions that you asked regarding how long to detox can be used when it comes to the question of detoxifying again.

My general answer is yes. You should detox at least once a year, depending on your lifestyle, work, toxic exposure, stress etc. Consider a six week detox once or twice a year; more often if you like. Understand that if you have been on the planet for 20, 30, 40, or more years, then your initial 8 or 12-week protocol may not be enough. Again, this is a very individual decision and a detox specialist such as myself can help you determine the correct path. For now, plan to revisit this process again next year. And, if you maintain a clean diet, you might even want to dig a bit deeper and consider the lemonade fast or a grape fast. You never know.

References

Campbell, T. C., & Campbell, T. M. (1968). The china study. Inter-University Consortium for Political Research.

Roy, M., Kiremidjian-Schumacher, L., Wishe, H. I., Cohen, M. W., & Stotzky, G. (1990). Selenium and immune cell functions. II. Effect on lymphocyte-mediated cytotoxicity. Experimental Biology and Medicine, 193(2), 143-148.

American Academy of Pediatrics Committee on Nutrition: The use of whole cow's milk in infancy. (1992). Pediatrics, (Jun), 89(6 pt 1), 1105-1109.

Postgraduate Medicine, 95, 115. (1994).

Journal of Dairy Science, 74(11), 4002-4012. (1991).

American Journal of Clinical Nutrition, 51, 489-489. (1990).

New England Journal of Medicine, 327(5), 302-307. (1992).

Lancet, 2, 66-71. (1989).

American Journal of Clinical Nutrition, 27(9), 916-925. (1974).

Gomm, W., von Holt, K., Thomé, F., Broich, K., Maier, W., Fink, A., ... & Haenisch, B. (2016). Association of Proton Pump Inhibitors With Risk of Dementia: A Pharmacoepidemiological Claims Data Analysis. *JAMA neurology.*

Iliff, J. J., Wang, M., Liao, Y., Plogg, B. A., Peng, W., Gundersen, G. A., ... & Nagelhus, E. A. (2012). A paravascular pathway facilitates CSF flow through the brain parenchyma and the clearance of interstitial solutes, including amyloid β. *Science translational medicine*, *4*(147), 147ra111-147ra111.

Xie, L. (2013). Sleep initiated fluid flux drives metabolite clearance from the adult brain. *Science.*

- Generally speaking, the body doesn't like isolates. It can have difficulty absorbing them (thus many individuals experience gas, bloating, or abdominal distress from the use of vitamins and minerals) and may consider them toxic if absorbed. As you would expect, the body prefers its vitamins and minerals bound to food—in their natural form, primarily bound to carbohydrates and some proteins. As a matter of fact, it is the small lipids, sugars, and amino acids attached to the vitamins and minerals that the individual cells of your body recognize and absorb, as opposed to the vitamins and minerals themselves. For the most part, naturally occurring vitamins and minerals just tag along for the ride into the cells. All things considered, there are important differences as to how different vitamins and minerals are absorbed.

CPSIA information can be obtained
at www.ICGtesting.com
Printed in the USA
LVHW04s0223100818
586597LV00021B/1686/P